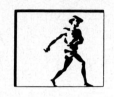

Jeff Aquilon & Nancy Donahue Aquilon

Photographs by BILL CONNORS

Exercise Consultant

Dr. JOSHUA SIMON, Columbia University

SIMON AND SCHUSTER   NEW YORK

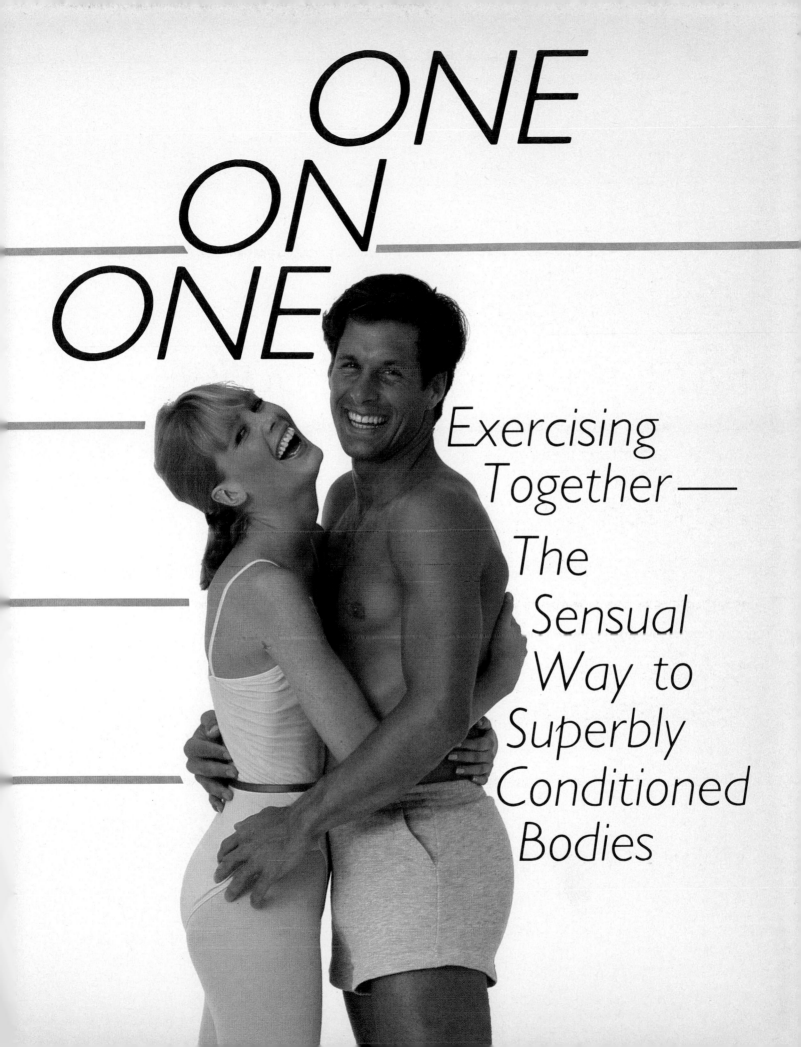

ONE ON ONE

Exercising Together— The Sensual Way to Superbly Conditioned Bodies

Published by Simon and Schuster
A Division of Simon & Schuster, Inc.
Simon & Schuster Building
Rockefeller Center
1230 Avenue of the Americas
New York, New York 10020
SIMON AND SCHUSTER and colophon are registered trademarks of Simon & Schuster, Inc.
Designed by Elizabeth Woll
Printed and bound in Italy.

10 9 8 7 6 5 4 3 2 1

Library of Congress Cataloging in Publication Data

Aquilon, Jeff.
   One on one.

   1. Isometric exercise.   2. Exercise.   3. Physical
fitness.   I. Aquilon, Nancy Donahue.   II. Title.
RA781.2.A584   1984   613.7′1   84-10664

ISBN: 0-671-50399-5

A Woodward/White Book

Kevin Dornan
Creative Director

G. Paul Hardin
Assistant Photographer

John Sommi
Zoli International

Juli Foster
Ford Model Management

Barbara Brehm
Consultant on Aerobic Exercise

The Casa Marina Resort Hotel
Key West, Florida

We want to give our special thanks to Danskin, Perry Ellis, Norma Kamali, Ralph Lauren, Mary Jane Marcasiano, Speedo, and Joan Vass for their clothing; to Bob Fink and Kerry Warn for hair styling, George Newell and Fran Cooper for makeup, and Daphne Wood for editorial assistance; to Vicki of Zoli International; to The Lighthouse Court, and The Oasis, Key West, Florida; to Connie Clausen, our agent; and to Bob Bender and Dan Green of Simon & Schuster.

For our families

CONTENTS

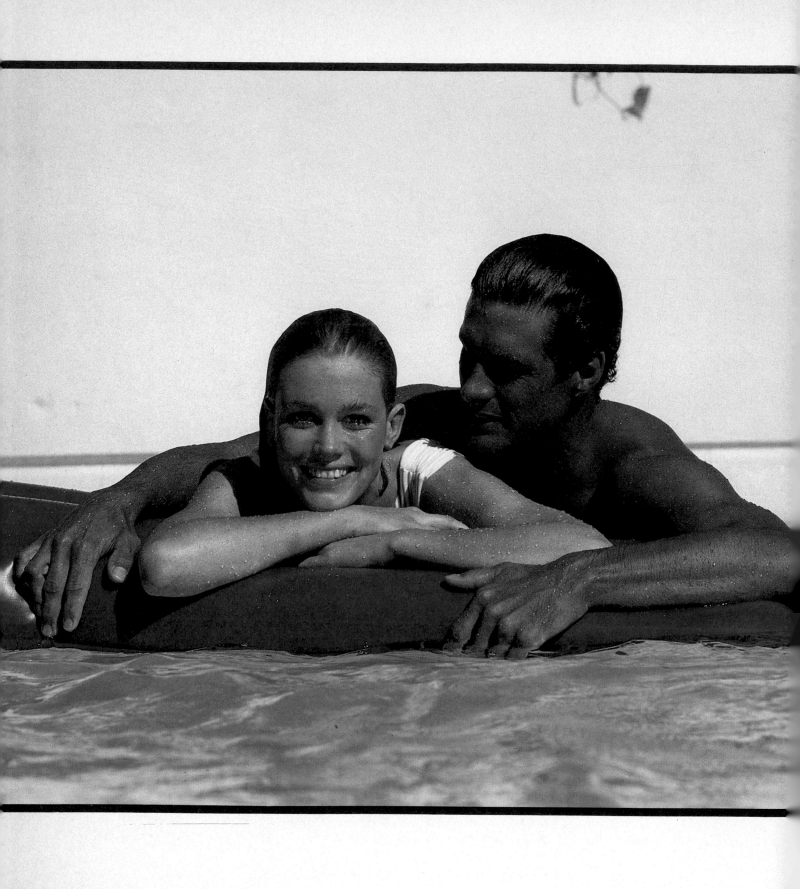

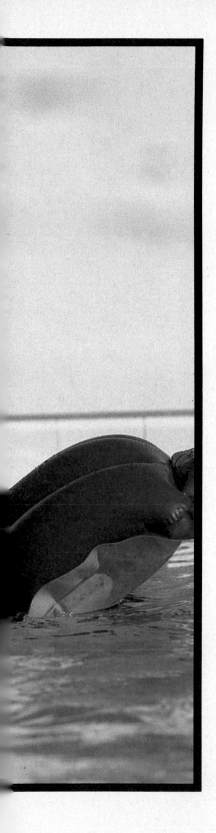

A SOUND HEART IN A SOUND BODY

Exercise can help you look good and feel terrific. No doubt about it. But there's more to being in shape than a sound body. Today, exercise is not just a form of self-improvement, it's a social opportunity. After two decades of sexual permissiveness, people are exploring other kinds of sensual experience, other ways to combine physical and emotional relationships. It's no coincidence that in most urban areas, gyms are replacing singles bars as the best place to meet someone.

To us exercise is not about self-gratification, it's about giving. It's about two people giving to each other, physically and emotionally, every day,

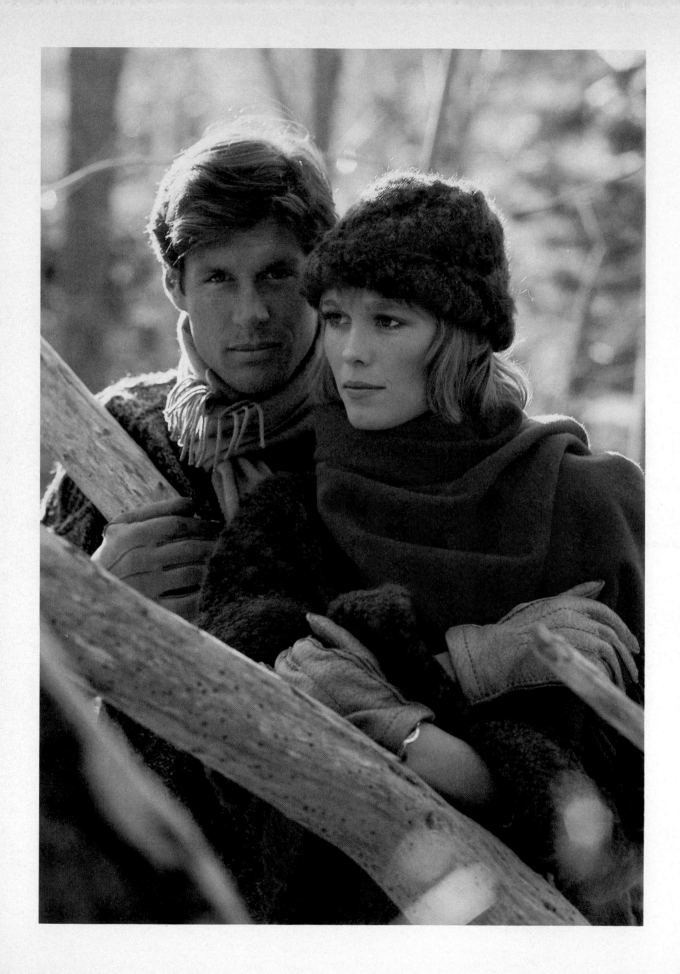

through keeping fit—being good to themselves and good to each other at the same time. The term "one on one" originally referred to two athletes squaring off against each other in practice. But to us it describes the feeling of intimate, mutual giving that comes from exercising together.

We believe each of us has an obligation to his or her own body, an obligation to treat it well, both physically and emotionally. We also believe we have an obligation to each other—to support each other, to care for each other, both emotionally and physically. Sometimes these obligations seem to be at odds, but they're not. You can't really take care of yourself without loving somebody else, and you can't fully love somebody else without taking care of yourself.

But, like millions of other two-career couples, we found that our time together was severely limited. Individual exercise routines—Jeff's trips to the health club and Nancy's aerobic sessions—were hours stolen from each other. The demands of our professional lives—frequent location shoots, high-pressure routines, and hectic working conditions—threatened our efforts to stay fit and our relationship.

We needed an approach to fitness that would allow us to maintain an exercise regimen and, at the same time, would strengthen the bond between us. We sought out a coed health club where we could work out together, and we developed a routine of exercises that would keep us both in top condition. Today, we incorporate this fitness program even into our rare moments of leisure at the end of the work day and on weekends at our home on Long Island where we swim, jog, and sail. Through exercise, we not only keep fit but also spend more time enjoying each other.

Many couples—from young roommates to couples with college-age children—find themselves in the same bind that we did. They have less and less time to divide among work, home, fitness, and being with each other. This book can change all that; it can give you back some lost time to enjoy yourself and to share with someone you love.

Millions of couples are looking for a way to be together more, to strengthen their relationship, to experience each other's lives more fully. This is what exercising together is all about: a sound heart in a sound body.

PUTTING FUN
INTO FITNESS

Unlike many models, we never really *decided* to go into modeling. We sort of fell into it. Jeff was captain of the water polo team at Pepperdine College in California when fashion photographer Bruce Weber happened to be on the West Coast looking for athletic "nonmodel" types. A few months later, a Weber photograph of Jeff appeared on the cover of *GQ*. Nancy was a college student who entered a cover-girl contest on a lark. A few months later, she was on the cover of *Mademoiselle*, and soon after on the cover of every major women's fashion magazine.

Up until that time, neither of us had been very "body-conscious." We were just who we were: a water polo jock from California and a pretty girl from Lowell, Massachusetts. We'd never *really* looked at ourselves in the mirror. As for pictures, we had the usual family snapshots and the usual reactions: "God, I look terrible." Like most people, neither of us felt particularly comfortable in front of a camera or particularly liked having our pictures taken.

Then—suddenly—we were both in New York (we hadn't met yet), caught in the whirlwind of the fashion industry, surrounded by people taking our pictures and talking about our bodies, seeing ourselves on magazine covers and in full-page newspaper advertisements. It was more than slightly unnerving.

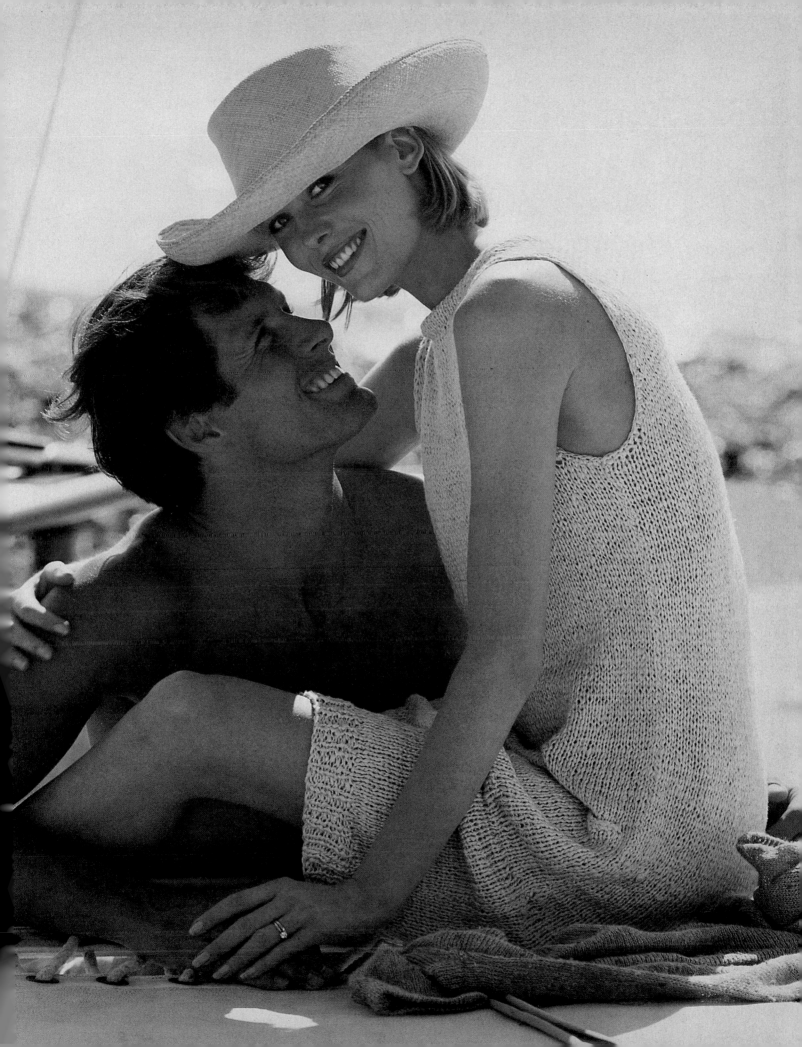

At first, we both tried to keep our new lives in perspective by ignoring the hoopla. As we went from studio to studio, from location to location, we tried to maintain the same carefree, unself-conscious attitude we had before being "discovered." We partied late, played hard, and seldom gave our bodies a second thought.

It wasn't until we met on a shoot and began to care about each other that we began to take a real interest in our own bodies. For the first time, we saw our bodies as assets—not just professional assets, but emotional and physical assets as well. Taking care of them was the least we could do, both for ourselves and for each other.

Nancy: Feeling Good About Yourself. Fitness was a watchword in my house for as long as I can remember. My mother was—and still is—the family coach and fitness guru. With eleven children, she needed to stay in good shape. At home, she converted our big basement into an exercise room and held classes three times a week for women in the neighborhood. At night, she taught a class in calisthenics for retarded children at the local YWCA.

But despite her busy schedule, my mother always found time at night for us to exercise together. Every single night, just the two of us would do an hour of calisthenics, jumping rope, and talking. That was the first place I learned that exercise is a good way to bring people closer together. All the time I was growing up, my mother and I were best friends, and I'm sure it's because we made a special place for each other every night in the basement workout area.

I still remember vividly the teenage trauma of buying a bathing suit. Like most of my girlfriends, I was unhappy with my body and buying a bathing suit meant facing up to all those insecurities. We all had different reasons for dreading the bathing-suit season. As for me, I hated my body because I was so thin and I would do anything to cover myself up. I was always the last one of my friends to stop bundling up in the spring, and the first one to start again in the fall. Even with boyfriends I was terrified to show myself, not because I was prudish, but just because I was afraid they would reject my skinny body.

When you're as thin as I was, going through high school and puberty at the same time is murder. It's no wonder I hated my body, or that I got so thin in the first place. When I was still very young my friends were always teasing me about the way I looked. They'd say, "You'll get fat," or "Watch out for those hips." Well, no way in the world was I going to let *that* happen. So I stopped eating and started exercising fanatically. Even though I was already thin, I was so afraid of getting fat that I starved myself even more. It didn't take long before my fat anxieties had turned into a mild case of anorexia. When I shrank to ninety-five pounds, my mother stepped in.

With her help, I began to eat and exercise more sensibly. But even when I won a contest to do the cover for *Mademoiselle* and went on to New York, I still wasn't really happy with myself. There I was, among all those beautiful, curvaceous women— skinny me. I wanted to exercise, but it wasn't easy. At first I skipped rope in my apartment. But without my mother there to exercise with me, it just wasn't the same. Pretty soon, I slacked off, and eventually I quit. I just didn't have the motivation to exercise regularly on my own. I joined a succession of gyms and health clubs (each friend had her own favorite). But I didn't want to go to a club after a long, hard day's work, I just wanted to go home and crash. Then Jeff and I hit on the idea of working out together. It was like being back in my basement at home.

I realized then that the more convenient you make your exercise, the easier it is to keep it up. It's also just plain *easier* if you're home doing your exercises *with* somebody. I'd taken that for granted during high school. I needed to come to New York to see how good I had had it in Lowell. Jeff and I motivate each other. When I was trying to exercise alone, it was much too easy to say, "All right, I've done enough of this." When we work out together, competition sets in and I say, "I can do as much as *he* can."

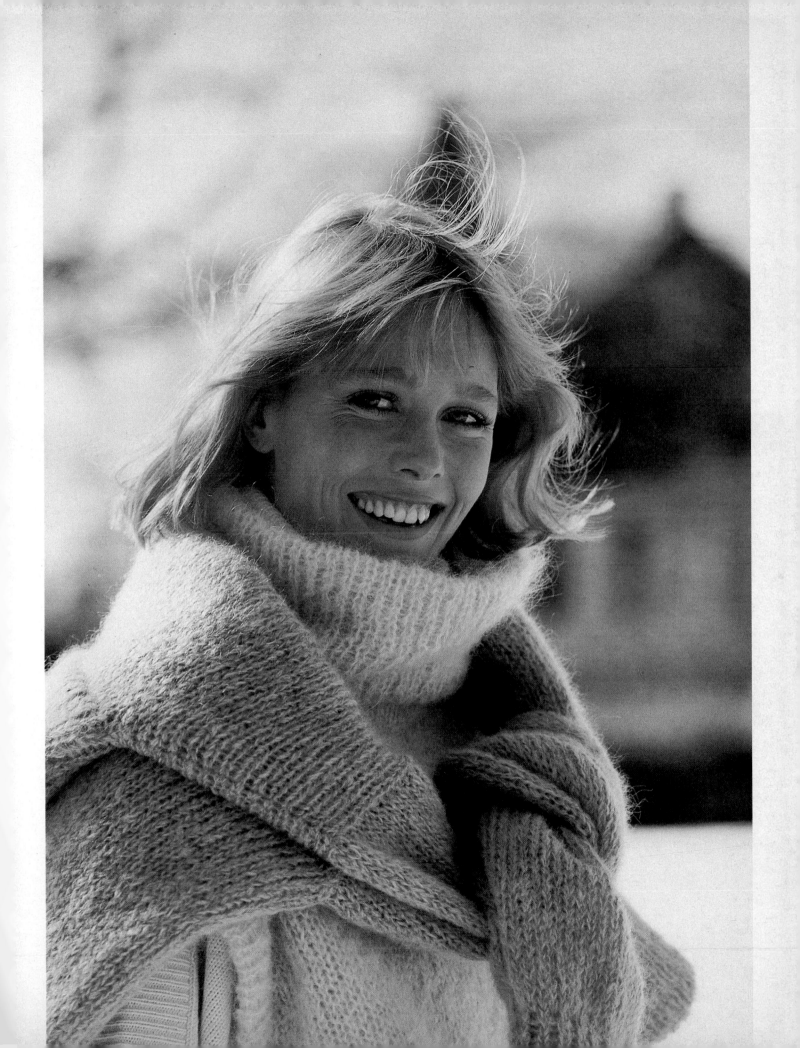

Today I feel confident about my body. I *like* the way I look. I'm convinced that exercising with someone gave me the combination of physical fitness and emotional support I needed to build my confidence in my own body and in myself. I also discovered that when you feel good about yourself, it's much easier for someone else to feel good about you.

Sometimes when Jeff is away on location and I have a few days off, I go home to visit my family. Whenever I do, my mother and I always exercise together. The last time I was home, we were down in the basement workout area, exercising, jumping rope, and talking. She said how great it was to have me home to exercise with again. No matter who you do it with, exercising is more fun if you do it together, but if you do it with the *right* people, it's the best.

Jeff: *"If It Feels Good, Do It."* Until I came to New York, my life was a California cliché. I started surfing when I was five years old and didn't quit until I came to New York. I loved the water so much, my parents couldn't pull me away from it. If the word got around that the swells were high on a school day, I would slip out and play hooky to catch them. I was always doing something—football, baseball, surfing, swimming, whatever—but I never thought of it as "exercise." It was just having a good time.

When high school came along, I had to think about exercise in a more systematic way for the first time. I had to choose a sport to go out for. Even though I'd been a water rat since diapers, I chose football. Don't ask me why. I suppose I was into the jock/ macho routine and wanted to prove myself on the playing field. Anyway, that didn't last very long. After getting knocked around for a few days, I realized that I belonged in the water. Besides, the football team used to run by the pool on the way to and from practices every day and I could see the swimmers (many of them old surfing buddies) lying by the pool and being cool. I thought, "This is work, that's for me."

I haven't forgotten that lesson. If exercise isn't fun, you won't enjoy it. If you don't enjoy it, you won't do it. So my first rule of fitness is: "If it feels good, do it." Pick something that's fun, something you can enjoy. Unless you're a diehard masochist (and I see them jogging around the city every day), that's the best insurance that you'll stick with it.

In high school, swimming was fun and that's what I did. Swimming eventually led to water polo, which I continued to play through college at Pepperdine. One reason I took to the water was that my father was also a swimmer. Whenever we talked, it was mostly about swimming. The water was our common ground, so to speak. Whenever possible, we would take off in his boat and sail to the channel islands. Like Nancy's mother, my father gave me the support and the confidence I needed to feel good about myself.

During college, I had no idea that I would end up as a model. My creative side wanted to be an architect. In high school I had worked as a landscape architect for the Los Padres National Forest Service designing picnic areas and comfort stations. No big deal, but an encouraging start. In college, my more practical side led me into business and computer sciences. Of course, I went back to the water when I could. During the summers, I took my old job as a lifeguard at the Santa Barbara beach, and during school I played water polo. One day, after an especially bruising game that left me with two black eyes, I bicycled over to meet some photographers from New York thinking, "What a waste of time." A few weeks later I was sitting in the offices of the Ford Modeling Agency in New York. I knew California had earthquakes, but I never expected one to strike in my life.

Unfortunately, my California lifestyle and my New York career didn't mix very well. You can't play hooky in Manhattan and run down to the beach. It's not easy even to swim regularly. I was used to going around in as few clothes as possible and East Coast winters came as a real shock. But the worst thing was that it was almost impossible for me to stick to my old rule, "If it feels good, do it." Exercise wasn't just "having fun" anymore, it was exercise. I

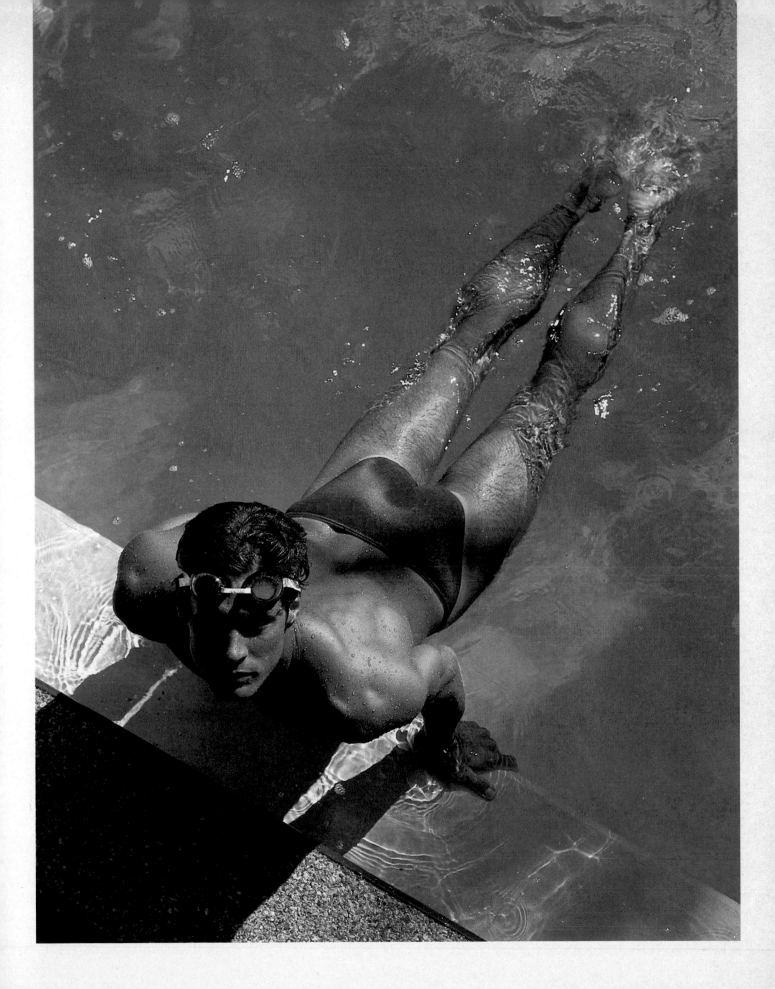

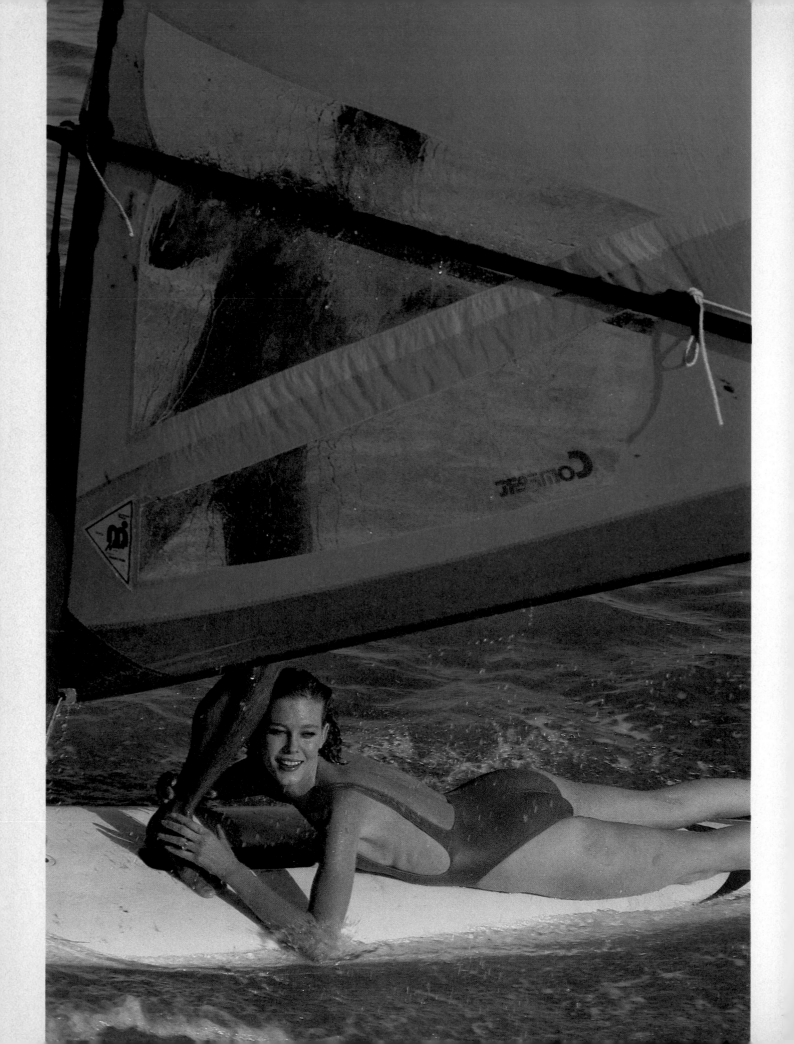

had to balance it with my busy working schedule, location trips, and the inhospitable weather. It probably would have been easier for me if I had developed an exercise regimen—the old "three times a week at the gym" routine. I could have transferred that more easily to my new life. But as it was, not being able to stay fit was really not being able to have fun.

For me, partner exercises put the fun back in fitness. No matter how bad the weather is or how busy my schedule, I look forward to time with Nancy for exercise. Whether we're downhill skiing (which Nancy is great at), wind-surfing (my new favorite), or doing our exercise routine, doing it together really does double the pleasure and makes exercise what it should be—fun.

UNLOCKING THE MOTIVATION DOOR

For both of us, as for most people, motivation was the problem with exercising regularly. It was the only thing that stood between us and real fitness.

We both had active childhoods, we both knew *how* to exercise and we both knew that we *should* exercise. What we needed was the motivation to change "I *want* to do it" into "I *will* do it."

Doing it together was, for us, the key that unlocked the motivation door. When that little voice inside says, "But it's so much trouble," or "I'm so tired" or "What's the point?" it makes all the difference to have somebody next to you answering in your other ear, "It's not trouble, it's fun"; or "I'm tired too, but let's do it anyway"; or "The point is that I love you and I want you to be the best you can be."

Our story may be unusual, but our situation—as a busy, two-career couple—is no different from that of millions of people who can't seem to find time for *both* themselves and the ones they love. You don't have to choose between your "selfish" need for personal fitness and your commitment to someone else. By learning to do it together, you can experience both the physical and the emotional satisfaction of being one on one.

DOING IT
TOGETHER

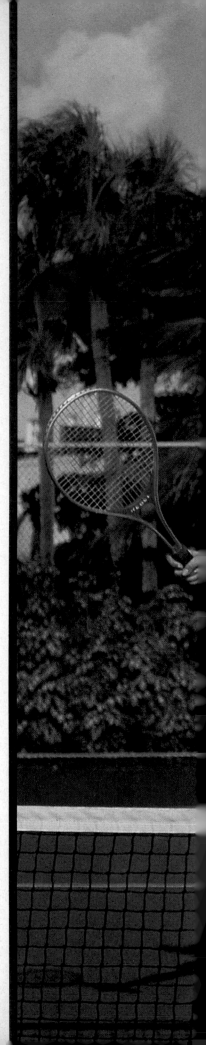

Doing it together means more than exercising at the same time in the same place. It means working closely with each other to make your exercise program better than any solo exercise program. Better because you'll each try to work harder, and better because exercising with your partner means you'll enjoy it more, so you'll do it more often and stay in better shape.

If you're a competitive person, exercising together can provide you with the encouragement you need to do better, and the consolation you need when you don't do as well as you want. By exercising together you can push each other to a level of exertion neither could achieve alone.

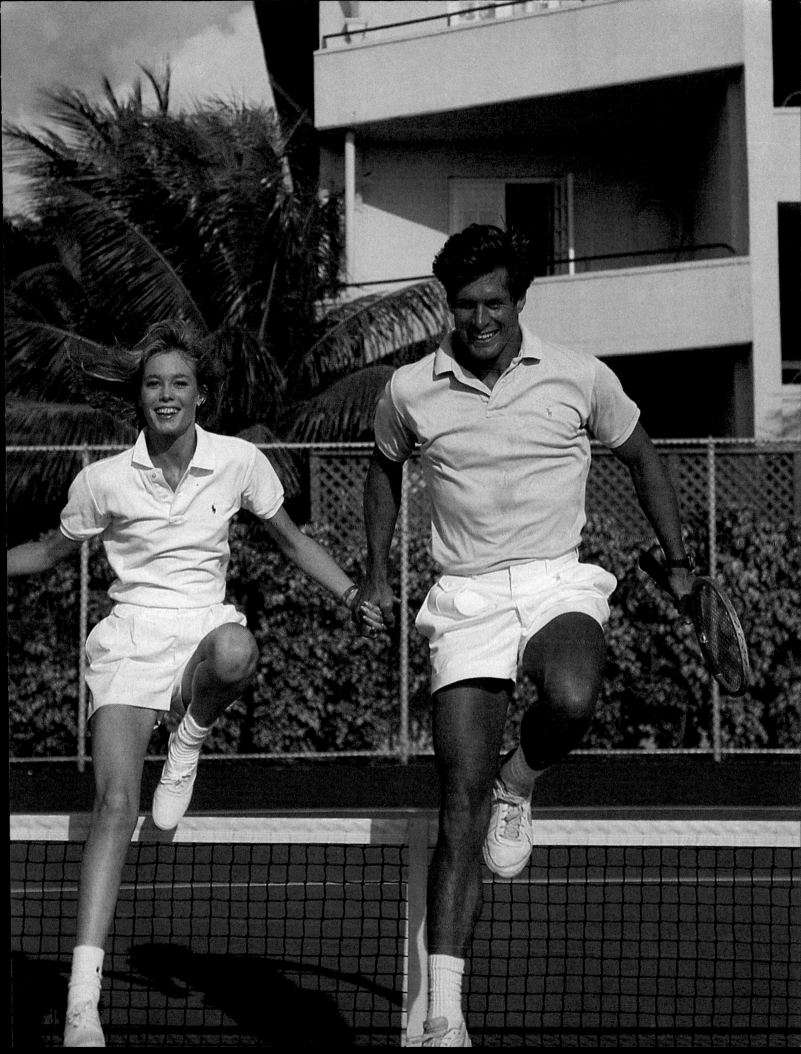

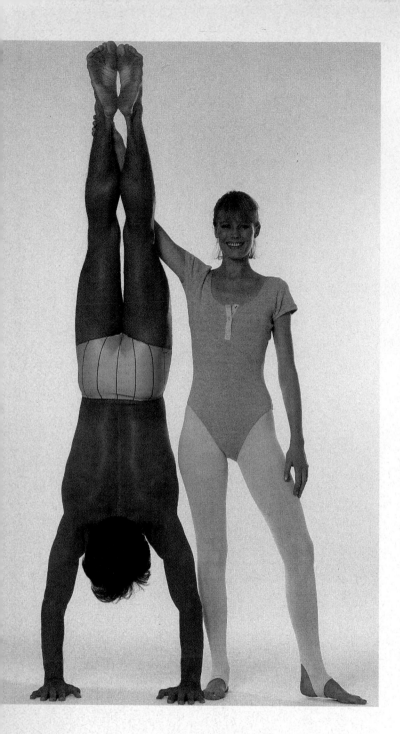

that feeling. Don't try to beat your best time, don't press. Just savor that feeling of control and motion.

This is especially important if you're a competitive person. Maybe what you need isn't a competitor, but someone to remind you to enjoy yourself. When we exercise together, we enjoy working at our upper limits every once in a while. Some days we want to beat our best time, or see who can do more repetitions. On those days, it's nice to have the other person there encouraging you to do your best. But most days, we just relax and go with the good feelings. Exercising together should bring joy, not pain.

MEN AND WOMEN'S BODIES: WORKING TOGETHER

When we began our One-on-One program, we faced the same problems most couples face. Physically, we seemed about as well matched as King Kong and Fay Wray. Jeff was a college athlete, bulging with muscles. He could lift Nancy with one hand. Nancy was slender and naturally fit, but, at 110 pounds, hardly up to a wrestling match. Because of our different body types, we were attracted to different kinds of exercise. Jeff swam endless laps when he could get to a pool while Nancy did her lonely aerobic routines off and on.

We wondered how we could possibly develop a regular exercise program that would allow for the differences in physique between us. First, we had to face the facts:

Men Are Stronger. As a general rule, at least, men have greater *muscular* strength. That's why men hold the records in all sports events that require exerting force against resistance—everything from shot-putting to swimming. A recent study at West Point concluded that women have, as a general rule, only about two-thirds the strength of men, based on a measurement of force per pound of body weight.

The biggest difference between men and women is in their upper bodies: Even compensating for

But exercising together doesn't have to be competitive—and most of the time it shouldn't be. You don't have to push yourself to the limit in order to benefit from exercise. There *is* gain without pain. Being physically fit is a good feeling and there are times when you should just go with

differences in body weight, men generally have much stronger arms and chests than women. When it comes to legs, however, the difference is very slight. Relative to body weight, women have about ninety percent of the strength of men in their leg muscles. If you account for the fact that more of a woman's weight is fat, and you compare strength per weight of muscle, women are actually slightly stronger in the legs than men.

The reason for men's superior muscle strength in the upper body is simply that men have more muscles. The hormone testosterone, which promotes the growth of muscle fibers, is present in much greater concentrations in men than in women. So even if a man and woman were to do the same rigorous program of strength exercises, the man would develop large muscles but the woman wouldn't.

Women Are More Flexible. Male muscle fibers also tend to be thicker than female muscle fibers, partly because men tend to use their muscles more often than women (use promotes thickness) and partly because men tend to neglect flexibility stretching even when they exercise actively. In fact, someone who is completely inactive will be more flexible than someone who works on developing strength but neglects flexibility. That's why women's muscles tend to be far more flexible than men's.

An exercise program for men and women to do together should take these differences into account. Too many workouts deal with these differences by trying to make a woman's body more like a man's. One of the great advantages of the One-on-One exercises is that you and your partner are in constant communication and therefore you can adjust to differences in height, strength, flexibility, and body type. After all, these are the same physical differences that enhance the act of making love. Why shouldn't they also enhance the act of exercising together?

Of course, it's possible to do any of these exercises with someone other than a spouse or someone of the opposite sex. On location shoots when we're apart, we both exercise with friends. In fact, for

exercises that require an approximate similarity in body weight, size, or strength, it can be preferable to do the exercises with a member of the same sex. That's why we chose to do some of the more difficult exercises with our friends John Sommi and Juli Foster (see pages 44 and 48). Ultimately, the only requirement for a partner in a One-on-One workout is that the two of you feel comfortable touching each other.

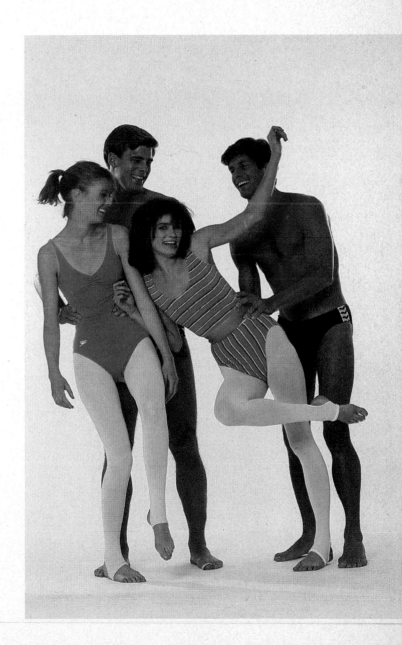

FIVE STEPS TO TOTAL FITNESS

What you want from any exercise program is *total fitness*. What good does it do you to run five miles every day if you can't open a drawer that's stuck? What's the point of having big biceps if you can't reach down to tie your shoes? Why work hard on toning your muscles if you feed your body junk? From the first, we wanted a fitness plan that would take care of all of our bodies' needs.

In putting such a plan together, we learned that there are five steps to real physical fitness:

- *Step One*:   FLEXIBILITY
- *Step Two*:   MUSCULAR STRENGTH
- *Step Three*: CARDIOVASCULAR ENDURANCE
- *Step Four*:   STRESS CONTROL
- *Step Five*:   NUTRITION

We set out to develop a routine of partner exercises that would incorporate all these elements in a program that was both fun and effective. We wanted it to be relatively easy to follow and not too time-consuming. Like a lot of couples, we have active careers and we don't want to spend all our time together on an exercise mat.

For us, the ideal fitness program is six days a week, forty-five minutes a day. Any less and you're cheating your health, any more and you'll come to resent it as a burden. Every workout starts with a flexibility warm-up of ten to fifteen minutes (pages 31–50). On the first, third, and fifth days, you should follow the warm-up with a set of isokinetic exercises for muscular strength lasting twenty to thirty minutes (pages 51–117). On the second, fourth, and sixth days follow instead with exercises

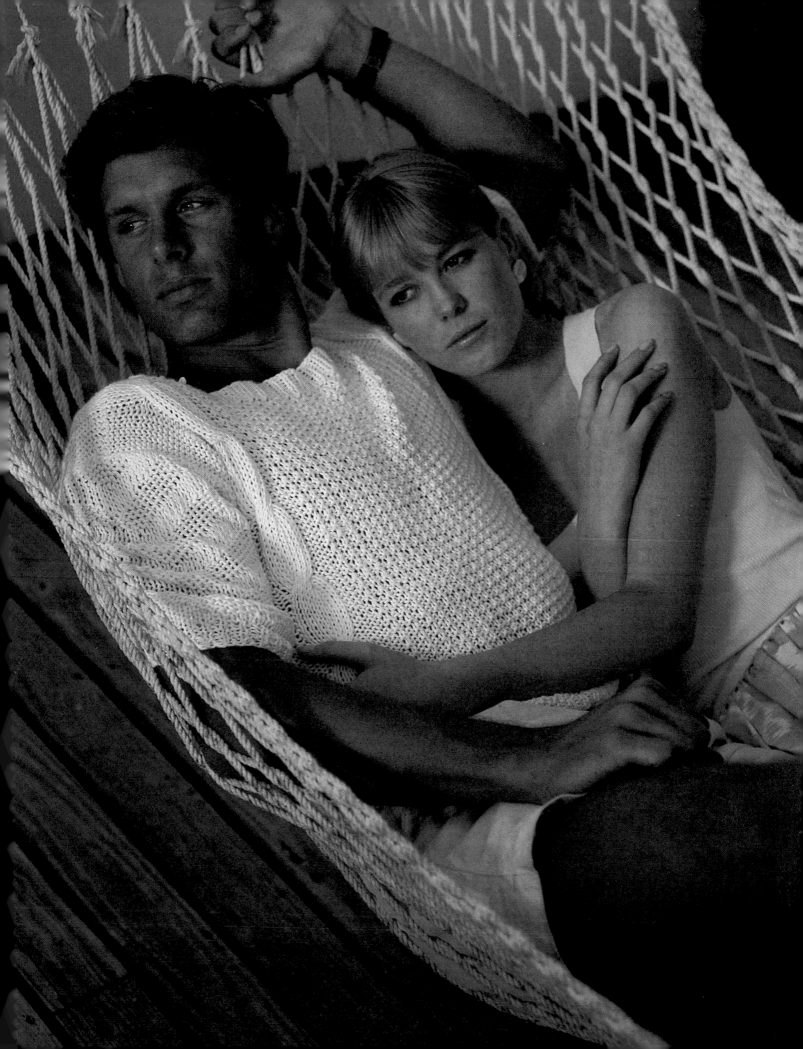

for cardiovascular endurance for about the same amount of time (pages 118–27). Every workout should end with a stress-control cool-down (pages 128–43) of ten or fifteen minutes.

We recommend following all the exercises in the order described. But we have organized the One-on-One program by muscle groups in the accompanying chart so you can see how comprehensive our workout is. Using the chart you can isolate and concentrate on exercises for specific parts of the body you want to work intensively.

As for nutrition (pages 144–51), we think of that as a six-day-a-week commitment too. We're only human; we like ice-cream too much. So we reserve one day every week when we can splurge. One of the joys of sticking to your routine of exercising together is that occasionally you can go out and eat something you shouldn't or spend a day doing nothing together. Sharing your occasional weaknesses can be as much fun as sharing your strengths.

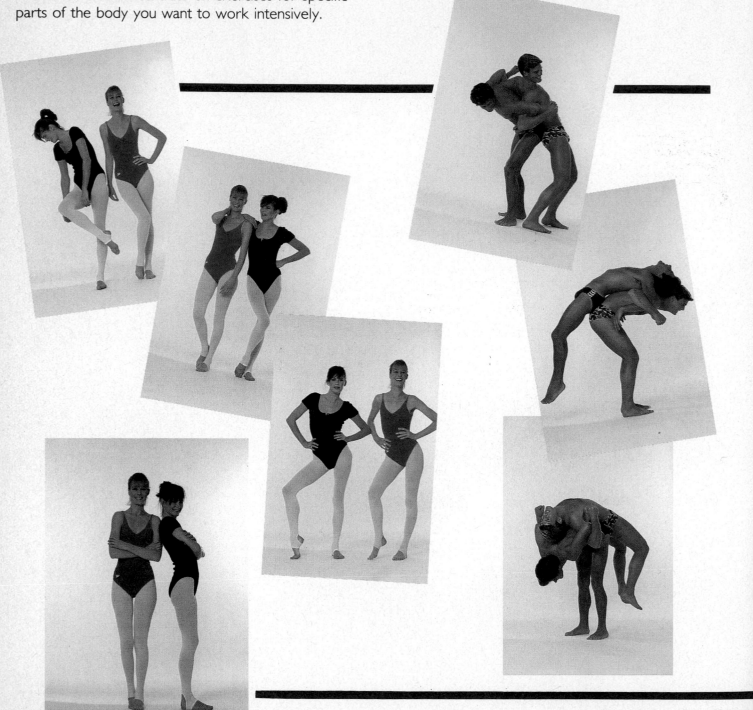

THE ONE-ON-ONE WORKOUT
A Muscle-by-Muscle Guide

Muscle Group	WARM-UP	ISOKINETIC	COOL-DOWN
Neck	III,3	II,5; IV,5	II,8
Shoulders	I,4	II,4; IV,1; VI, 1,2; VII,1,2	I,2; II,1,3,8
Arms	III,1,2; IV,1,2,3,4	I,3; IV,1,2,3; V,1,2,3,4	I,2
Chest	I,4; III,1	II,4; IV,3; VI,1,2; VII,1,2	II,1,3
Back	I,1; II,1	I,3,4; IV,2	I,1; II,6,8
Abdomen	I,3; II,1	I,2; IV,4; IX, 1,2,3	I,1
Buttocks	I,1	I,2; II,1; VIII,1,2,3,4	II,4
Hips	I,2; II,1; V,1,2,3	II,1,2; VIII,1,2,3,4	I,1,II,2,4,5
Thighs	I,2; II,4; V,1,2,3	II,2; VIII,1,2,3,4	II,2,4,5,6
Hamstrings	II,4	II,2,3	II,5,7
Calves	II,2,3	I,1; III,1	
Ankles	II,2,3	I,1	

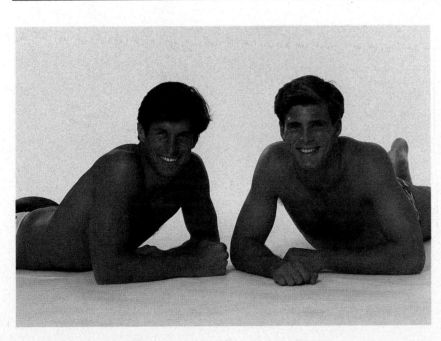

STEP ONE/*Flexibility*

THE WARM-UP

I t's hard to exaggerate the importance of warming up before exercising. Stretching increases the elasticity of your muscles and tendons, which makes a strain or pull less likely and gives you a freer range of motion while you're exercising. By increasing blood circulation and raising body temperature, stretching prepares your body for the heightened metabolic activity (quick conversion of food to energy) of strength and endurance routines.

Jeff: A Special Problem for Men. I learned how important stretching is when I was swimming on the Pepperdine water polo team. I learned the hard way. I had little patience for warm-ups then, so I skimmed through them and hit the pool going a hundred miles an hour. As a result, I damaged my shoulder muscles permanently.

Nancy doesn't have this problem because her muscles are more lithe and flexible than mine. She can reach down and put her palms on the floor as soon as she gets up in the morning. I have to work at it for a while. A lot of women are as limber as Nancy—or they can get that way without too much work. Men, on the other hand, even if they're in good shape, tend to have flexibility problems.

That's why I suggest that men work extra hard during the warm-up. You don't have to stretch for an hour if you're just jogging a few times around the block, but you do need to be careful. Going at anything hard, whether it's isokinetic exercises or helping the neighbors move their furniture, can be downright dangerous if you don't stretch out.

Flexibility is one reason I don't like weight-lifting. Lifting weights tightens and bulks up your muscles more than most exercises. A lot of male models have pumped themselves up so big they can't wear normal clothes anymore. That's a serious problem in a job where you're changing clothes all day. But it's uncomfortable and unnecessary for anybody. Of course, *any* exercise tightens up your muscles to some extent, but always gear your warm-up to your workout: The harder you exercise, the longer you should stretch.

Gain Without Pain. Stretching should *not* be painful. It may involve some discomfort if you're out of shape, but it should never be painful. If you experience pain you're *over*stretching.

People tend to overstretch because they're able to do it. They can stretch farther than they should, so they do. Flexibility should come gradually because you're really changing the elasticity of your muscles and their tendons. If you stretch out well six times a week, as we recommend, you won't notice a big improvement day by day. But the improvement will come. After a week or so, you'll be able to hold a position for twenty seconds that would have been painful when you started.

A lot of people have been brainwashed into thinking that "there's no gain without pain" so they resist the idea that exercise, in any form, can be enjoyable. Forget that stuff. Pain is your body's way of saying you're pushing too far. Tired, yes; out of breath, yes; but in pain, no.

Exercising together is particularly important in the warm-up. When you try to stretch fully a muscle or muscle group by yourself, often you will tend to tense the muscles you're trying to stretch. But tensing is the *opposite* of stretching. So you end up working against yourself. With a partner, you don't have to tense up at all and you gain the full benefit of the stretch in a way that's simply impossible by yourself.

One final word: Don't bounce. Recent studies have shown that you can damage a muscle by bouncing in a stretched position. Instead, stretch your partner as far as he or she is comfortable, hold that extended position for ten to twenty seconds, then let the muscle release completely before repeating.

WARM-UP EXERCISES

The warm-up routine should be done every day before any muscular strength or cardiovascular endurance routine.

- Duration: Ten to fifteen minutes.
- Order: Sequences I–III, as follows.
- Repetitions: Two or three per exercise (each position, each partner) equals one set. Beginners and intermediates, do one set; advanced, two (four to six repetitions total).

SEQUENCE 1 *Starting Position*

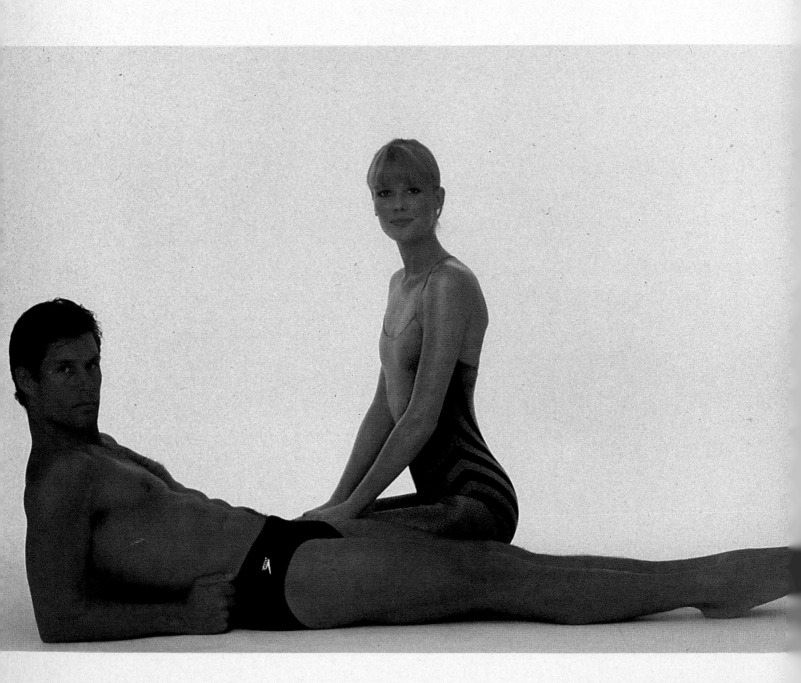

SEQUENCE 1   *#1 lower back, buttocks*

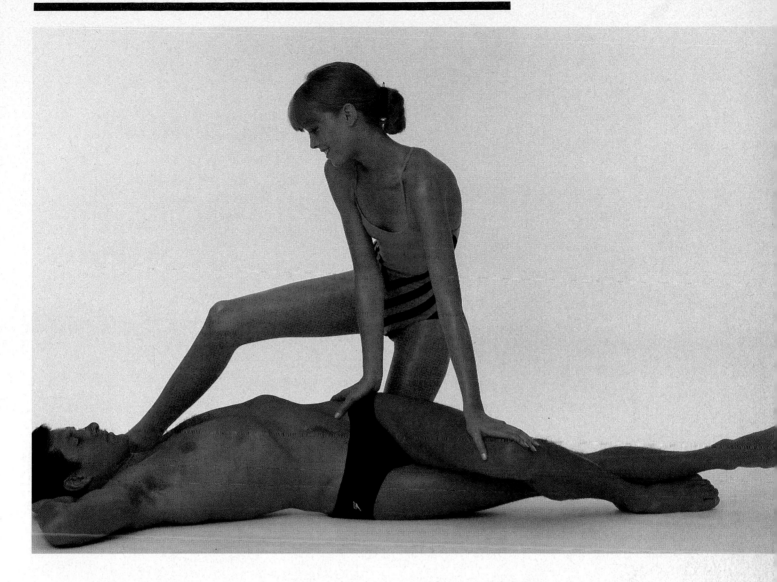

In these exercises, the "passive partner" (the person being stretched) should relax as much as possible. The "active partner" (the one who applies pressure) controls the exercise but should always be sensitive to the passive partner's responses.

PASSIVE PARTNER:

Lie back, put your hands behind your head, bend your knees slightly, and cross your legs. Secure the top leg by tucking the foot under the opposite calf. Relax as your partner performs the stretch.

ACTIVE PARTNER:

Rotate your partner's lower body by pushing at the knee and lifting at the hip. Go slowly at first. To get the best stretch, your partner's elbow on your side should stay on the floor. Put your foot on it to make sure it does. Watch your partner to know when he's had enough. Repeat on the other side with the other leg.

Both partners remain in the same positions for the next exercise.

SEQUENCE I *#2 hips, thighs*

PASSIVE PARTNER:

Arms at your sides, raise one leg to a comfortable height, keeping it straight at the knee. After one leg is stretched, lower it so that your partner is between your legs and can more easily repeat the exercise on the other leg.

ACTIVE PARTNER:

Continue to raise your partner's leg by lifting at the ankle. Once the leg is past perpendicular (if it goes that far), push the heel from behind. At the same time, help keep the leg straight by placing one hand just above the knee and pushing back. For maximum stretch, the leg you're not working with should stay on the floor. Anchor it with your foot or knee if necessary. Repeat with the other leg.

Passive partner, roll over.

SEQUENCE I *#3 abdomen, spine alignment*

PASSIVE PARTNER:

Prop your upper body on your elbows. (For stability, keep your elbows bent at right angles as shown.) Don't "hunch" your shoulders.

ACTIVE PARTNER:

Kneel and straddle your partner. Apply pressure through the heels of your hands on each side of the spine. Let up a little when your partner inhales; increase the pressure when he exhales. Whisper "breathe" to your partner to keep the timing right. Don't apply too much pressure in this exercise, especially if you're significantly heavier than your partner. If your partner feels discomfort (most likely in the lower back) you're leaning too heavily. Ease up.

Remain in the same positions.

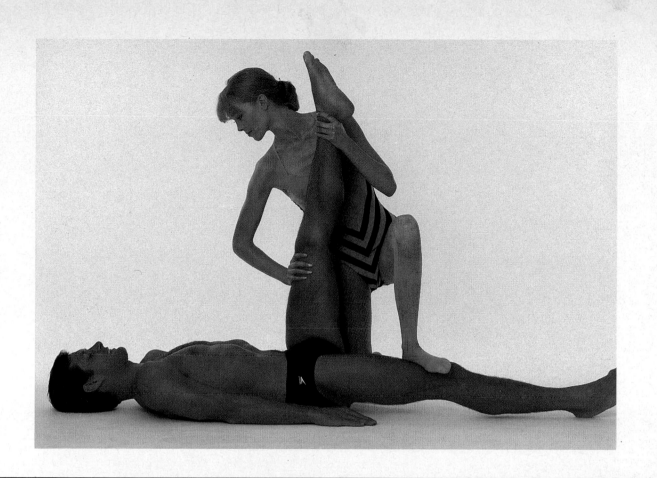

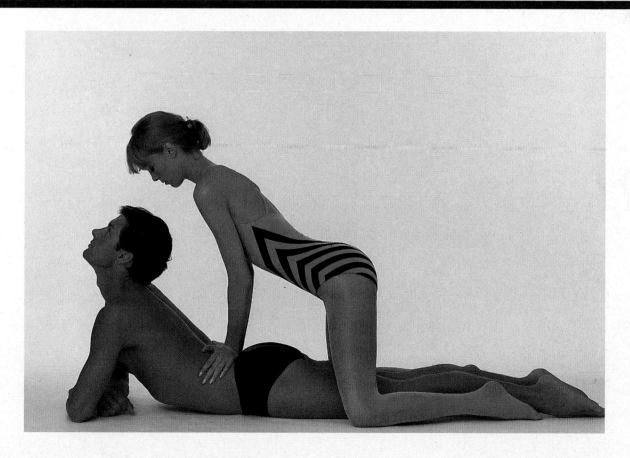

SEQUENCE I   *#4 shoulders, chest*

PASSIVE PARTNER:

Prop your upper body on your elbows as in the previous exercise. Remember not to hunch your shoulders.

ACTIVE PARTNER:

Kneel on one side of your partner. This time one hand should be on top of the other, only the heel of the top hand applying pressure on your partner's upper spine. Repeat several times at different spots on the upper back if you like, coordinating your pressure with your partner's breathing as before. Again, watch for signs of discomfort and don't overdo it.

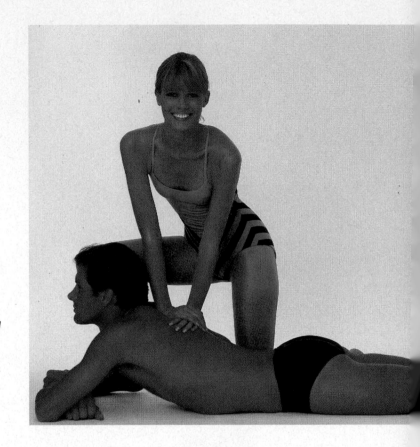

Go back to the beginning of Sequence I and switch positions.

SEQUENCE II *Starting Position*

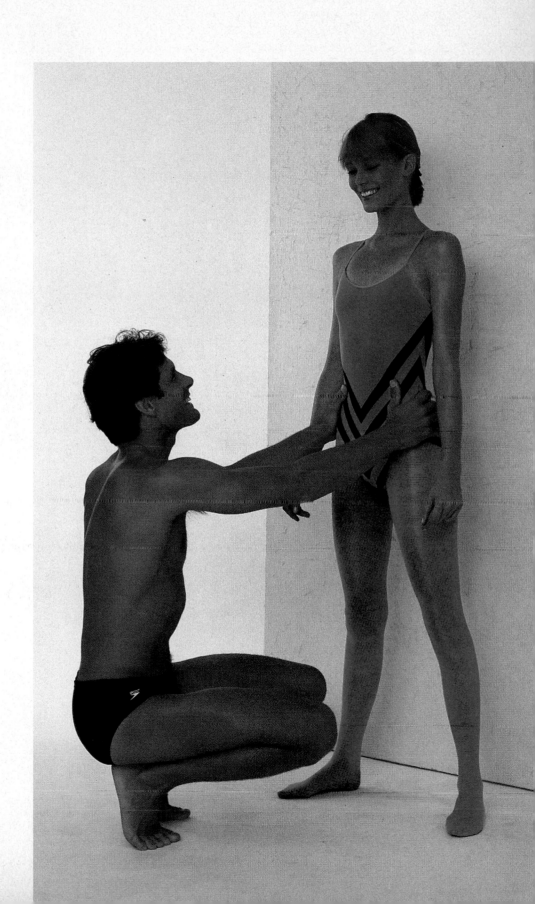

SEQUENCE II

#1 back,
abdomen, hips

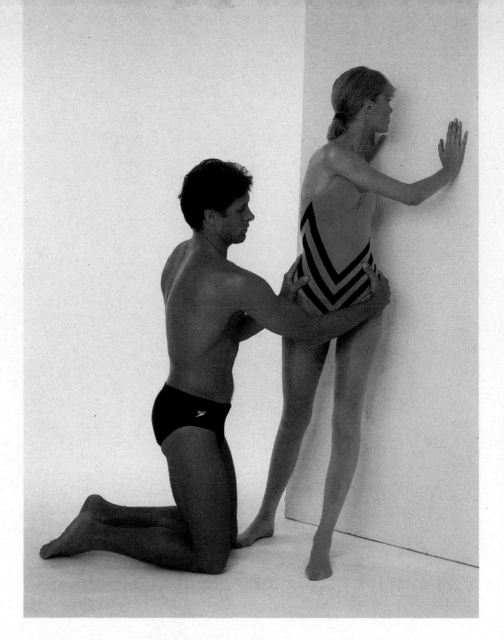

PASSIVE PARTNER:

Without moving your feet, turn your upper body until you're facing the wall behind you. Put your palms against the wall at shoulder height and about shoulder width apart. Throughout the exercise, keep your feet and hands firmly planted and your face toward the wall. After one side is stretched, turn all the way around without moving your feet, and face the wall over the opposite shoulder so the other side can be stretched.

ACTIVE PARTNER:

Turn your partner's midsection slowly toward the front by placing your hands on his or her hips and rotating the pelvis forward. Keep the pressure equal on both hips. Stop if your partner complains of pain.

Active partner goes down on both knees.

SEQUENCE II

#2 calves, lower legs

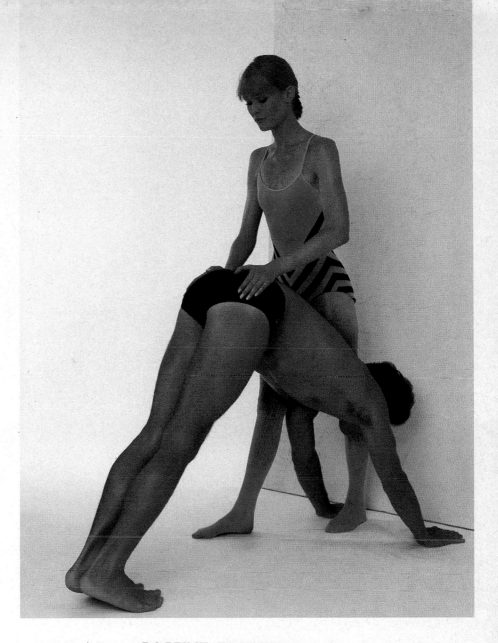

In the other exercises in this sequence, the passive partner is being stretched, and the active partner is applying the pressure. In this stretch, however, the active partner is being stretched and the passive partner is assisting the stretch. We have inserted this exercise here to improve the flow of the routine.

ACTIVE PARTNER:

Put your hands, about shoulder width apart, so your fingers just touch the wall behind your partner's feet. With your legs together, raise yourself up into the "bridge" position shown. Keep your knees and elbows straight; hands and feet firmly planted.

PASSIVE PARTNER:

Step forward and lean your thigh against the middle of your partner's back. For stability, put your hands on his or her buttocks. Make sure that you're leaning on your thigh, not the point of your knee. Gradually—very gradually because the stretching sensation here can be acute—lean more of your weight against the back.

Active partner, stand up. Passive partner, put your feet together and your back against the wall.

SEQUENCE II #3* calves, lower legs

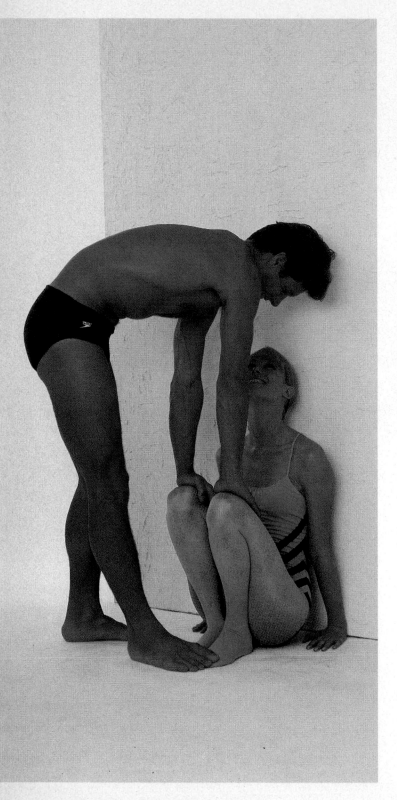

PASSIVE PARTNER:

Keeping your knees together and your feet close to the wall, slide down to a seated position as shown. Your buttocks and back should be straight and flat against the wall, and your heels on the floor. Relax.

ACTIVE PARTNER:

Lean down on your partner's knees, pushing them forward and down. Don't expect a great deal of movement if you're just beginning, and don't force extra movement. Always keep a sharp eye for signs of your partner's discomfort.

Both partners, remain in the same positions.

*This exercise may be substituted if the preceding one is too difficult.

SEQUENCE II *#4 hamstrings, thighs*

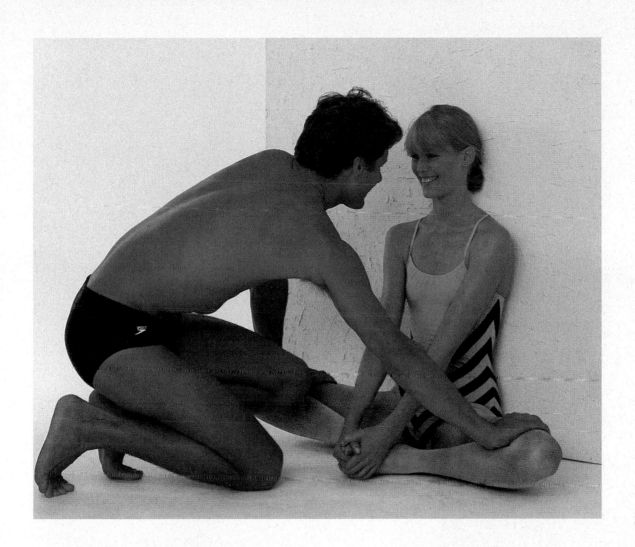

PASSIVE PARTNER:

Pull your feet up as close to your groin as possible, place them sole-to-sole, and hold them there. Keep your buttocks and back straight and flat against the wall. This is one exercise where people often subconsciously resist the stretch; they refuse to let go and relax. Fight the "uptightness" by thinking of your knees as heavy weights sinking slowly toward the floor.

ACTIVE PARTNER:

Put your hands on the insides of your partner's legs and slowly lean your weight down, pushing her knees toward the floor. Make sure you apply the same pressure on both legs and maintain your own balance.

Go back to the beginning of Sequence II and switch positions.

SEQUENCE III

Starting Position

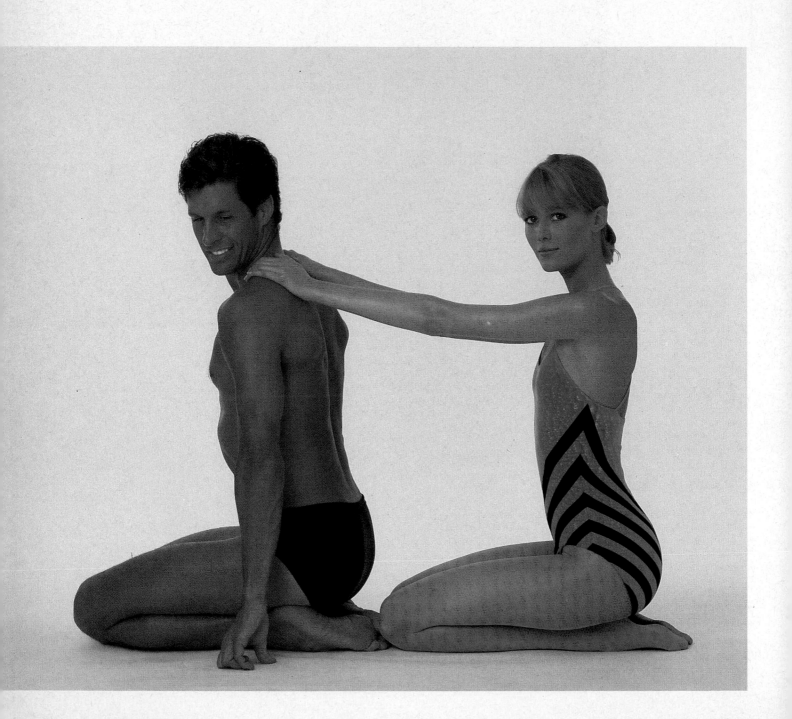

SEQUENCE III   *#1 arms, chest*

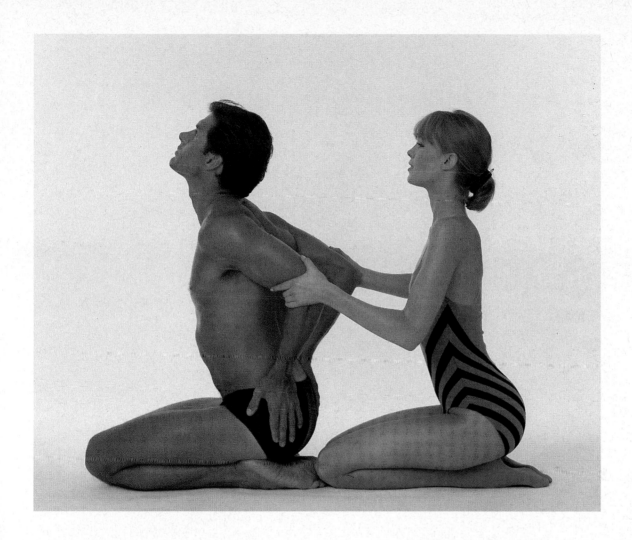

PASSIVE PARTNER:

Put your hands on your hips, fingers pointing down, and don't allow them to move. Keep your back straight and relax (don't hunch those shoulders).

ACTIVE PARTNER:

Slowly bring your partner's elbows back and toward each other. Be firm—these are tight, tough muscles—but not too firm. It isn't necessary for the elbows to touch, so don't force them.

Passive partner, stretch your legs out, and lie face-up with your head at your partner's knees.

SEQUENCE III *#2 arms*

PASSIVE PARTNER:

Prop yourself up on your arms. Keep your elbows straight and place your hands as far behind you as you comfortably can, shoulder-width apart.

ACTIVE PARTNER:

Kneel behind your partner. Grip his wrists and gradually slide his hands toward you, as shown, keeping them shoulder-width apart at all times. Make sure the elbows stay straight and the shoulders stay down. This can be an acute stretch, so watch for signs of discomfort.

Active partner, shift to a sitting position, legs apart. Passive partner, lay your head back between your partner's legs.

SEQUENCE III *#3 neck*

PASSIVE PARTNER:

Lie back. Put your arms down at your side, bring your knees up, and relax as totally as you can. Close your eyes.

ACTIVE PARTNER:

Sit behind your partner. Ease up close enough so you can cradle your partner's head in your hands. Anchor your partner's shoulders by pressing them gently down with the balls of your feet. Holding the head gently but firmly, lift it upward and forward.

Of all the stretches, this one should be done with the most care. For most people, the neck is a storehouse of tension. But it's also one of the body's most sensitive muscle groups. You will probably feel the tension as you ease the head forward and the chin nears the chest. If you or your partner sense resistance, hold the head in that position. If the resistance dissolves, continue the exercise slowly. If it doesn't, ease your partner's head gently back down.

Go back to the beginning of Sequence III and switch positions.

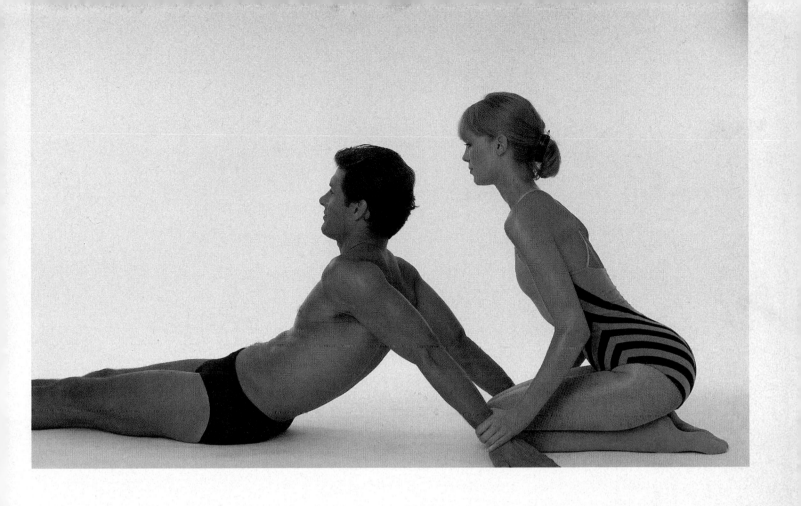

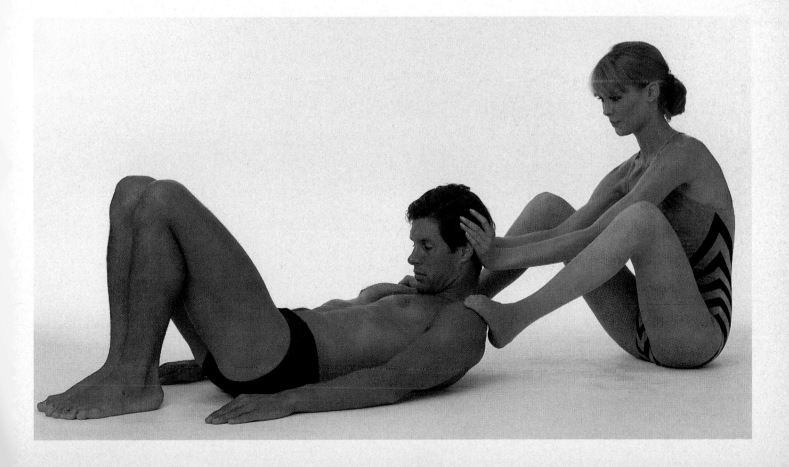

SPOT STRETCHES

Some people need special work on certain muscle groups, either because those muscles are used extensively or because they've fallen into disuse. There are also cosmetic reasons for working harder on some areas of the body than on others. Men may want to build up their arms and chest while women may want to tone down their hips and thighs.

With this in mind, we've included here some additional flexibility exercises so you can adjust your exercise program to meet your own special needs. We want to thank fellow models and friends Juli Foster and John Sommi for demonstrating these exercises with us, and for helping us show that exercising together can complement any kind of relationship.

SPOT STRETCHES FOR ARMS

Begin your workout by adding at least one additional set of the following stretches from the warm-up: III,1; III,2.

When you feel comfortable, unchallenged, or just bored with repeating those stretches, add the following sequence to your workout. These stretches can be done separately or they can be substituted for Sequence III,2 in the warm-up:

SEQUENCE IV #1

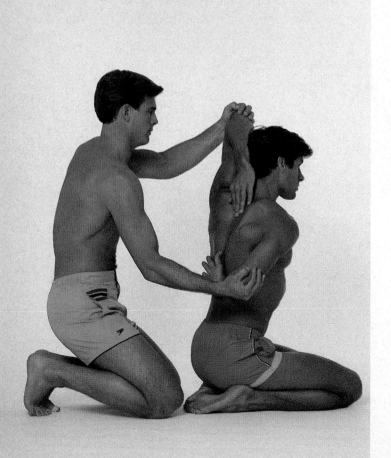

PASSIVE PARTNER:

Sit on your feet, as shown. With one arm, reach behind your head as far as you can with your elbow pointing straight up. With the other arm, reach behind your shoulder so that the elbow is pointing straight down. Try to lock your fingers about at the level of your shoulder blades. If you can't, reach as close as you can, but don't arch your back in the effort to make contact. Repeat the exercise, reversing the positions of your arms.

ACTIVE PARTNER:

Kneel behind your partner. Grasp your partner's elbows. If his hands reach far enough to link, gradually draw the elbows toward you. If they don't, try to bring them closer together by pulling up on the forearm of the lower arm and pushing down on the elbow of the upper arm.

Remain in the same positions.

SEQUENCE IV *#2*

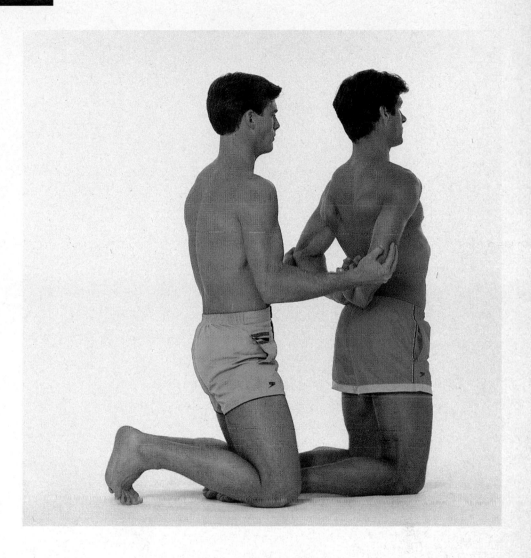

PASSIVE PARTNER:

Kneeling upright this time, maintain the same straight stance, making sure your back and head are in a straight, perpendicular line. Clasp your hands behind your back, fingers interlocked. The hands should be as high as possible and the palms touching.

ACTIVE PARTNER:

You may need to help your partner assume the correct position. If so, that effort will probably be a sufficient stretch. If your partner can reach the position unassisted, grasp his elbows and bring them slowly toward you and closer together.

Face each other on your knees.

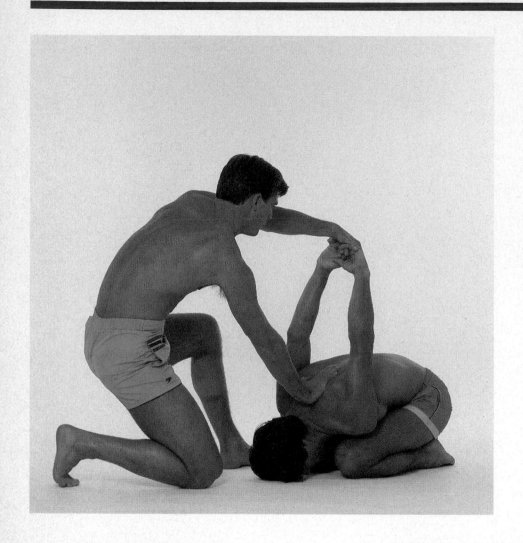

PASSIVE PARTNER:

Sit on your feet, as shown. Bend at the waist until your forehead touches the floor just at your partner's knees. Extend your arms behind your back and lock your hands. Your arms should remain straight throughout the exercise.

ACTIVE PARTNER:

Place one hand squarely and firmly in the middle of your partner's back, between the shoulder blades. With the other hand, grasp your partner's locked hands and slowly bring his arms toward you. The motion will be forward and upward. Maintain pressure on the back to prevent your partner's upper body from rising as you pull. The range of motion may be very limited, so go slowly and watch your partner's responses closely.

Passive partner, turn and face away from your partner, remaining on your knees.

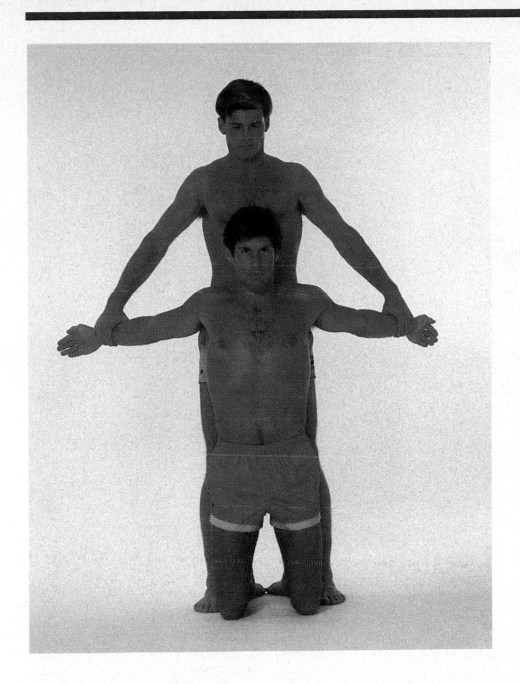

PASSIVE PARTNER:

Stretch your arms out and back as far as you can, as shown, keeping your palms facing out, your elbows straight, and your shoulders relaxed.

ACTIVE PARTNER:

Grip your partner's arms at the wrists and pull them slowly backward. For additional leverage, you can prop your knee against your partner's back. Proceed with care until your partner signals you to stop.

If you wish, go back to the beginning of the sequence and switch positions.

SPOT STRETCHES FOR THIGHS AND HIPS

Begin your workout by adding at least one additional set of the following stretches from the warm-up: I,1; I,2; II,4. The following stretches can be done in addition to these three exercises, or instead of them.

SEQUENCE V #1

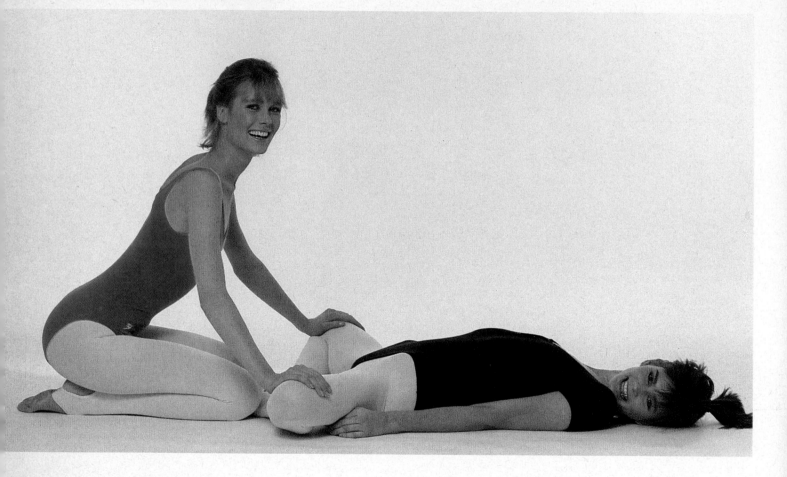

PASSIVE PARTNER:

Lie back and put your arms down at your sides. Bring your feet up as close to your buttocks as possible. Now spread your knees apart and put the soles of your feet together. Let your knees drop as far as they will go without letting your feet slide away from your buttocks. Keep your lower back pressed against the floor.

ACTIVE PARTNER:

Sit on your feet in front of your partner, as shown. Place your hands on the insides of your partner's knees and very slowly lean your weight downward. You can prevent the feet from sliding away from the buttocks by bracing them with your knees. Keep your arms straight and direct the pressure straight downward.

Remain in the same positions.

SEQUENCE V *#2*

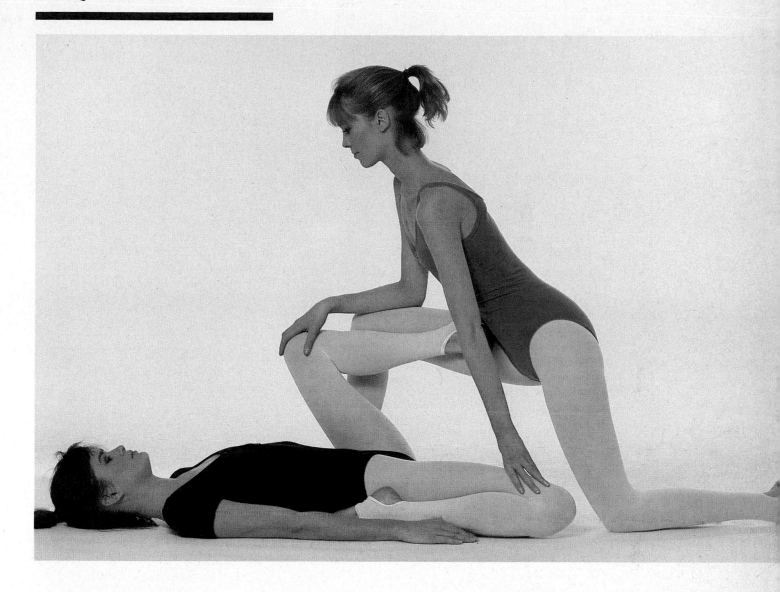

PASSIVE PARTNER:

Lying on your back, bring one foot up under your buttocks, keeping the knee pointed straight down. Bend the other leg up and place your foot against your partner's side just above the thigh. You should feel the stretch in the leg that's down. Repeat on the other leg.

ACTIVE PARTNER:

Secure the knee that is down with one hand. Stabilize the leg that is up with your other hand and the inside of your thigh, as shown. Gradually lean forward, pushing the knee of the upper leg toward your partner's chest. Move to the opposite side and repeat the stretch with the other leg.

Remain in the same positions.

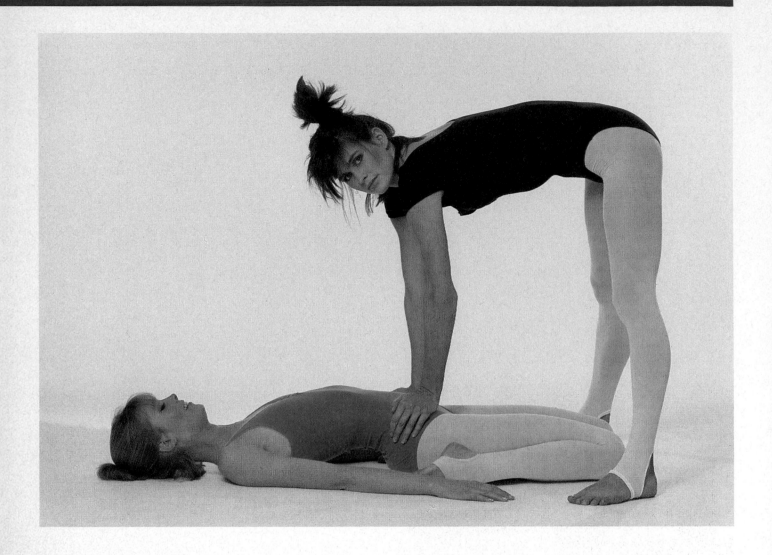

PASSIVE PARTNER:

Bend your knees and bring both feet up until your heels are tucked under your buttocks as in the previous exercise. Your knees should be together and pointing downward. Ask your partner to help you assume the appropriate position if necessary.

ACTIVE PARTNER:

Stand up, lean over and place your hands on your partner's hip bones. Lean your weight gradually onto them. The most important thing is to apply pressure evenly on both hips. You can use your legs to keep your partner's legs close together. This stretch can produce some acute sensations, so go slowly.

If you wish, go back to the beginning of the sequence and switch positions.

STEP TWO/*Muscular Strength*

ISOKINETICS

Muscles develop strength and endurance as a result of being exerted against resistance, or "overloaded." If the overload is sufficiently intense and long-lasting, it will cause the muscles to adapt—that is, to enlarge. Although most people find a well-tuned body attractive, the advantages go far beyond cosmetics. By toning the body's muscles you protect your joints and organs and prevent the nagging muscular aches and pains that afflict so many people. You're also better able to handle daily routines, weekend activity, and emergency exertion.

ISOKINETICS

When we started to develop an exercise routine that would improve muscular strength for *both* of us, we ran into problems. Weight-lifting was out because we needed a room full of expensive equipment and because we spent half our time in the weightroom adjusting the weights. Besides, spotting for your partner doesn't really involve both of you in the exercise. Isometrics didn't work either, because Jeff was so much stronger.

After consulting experts, we finally found what we

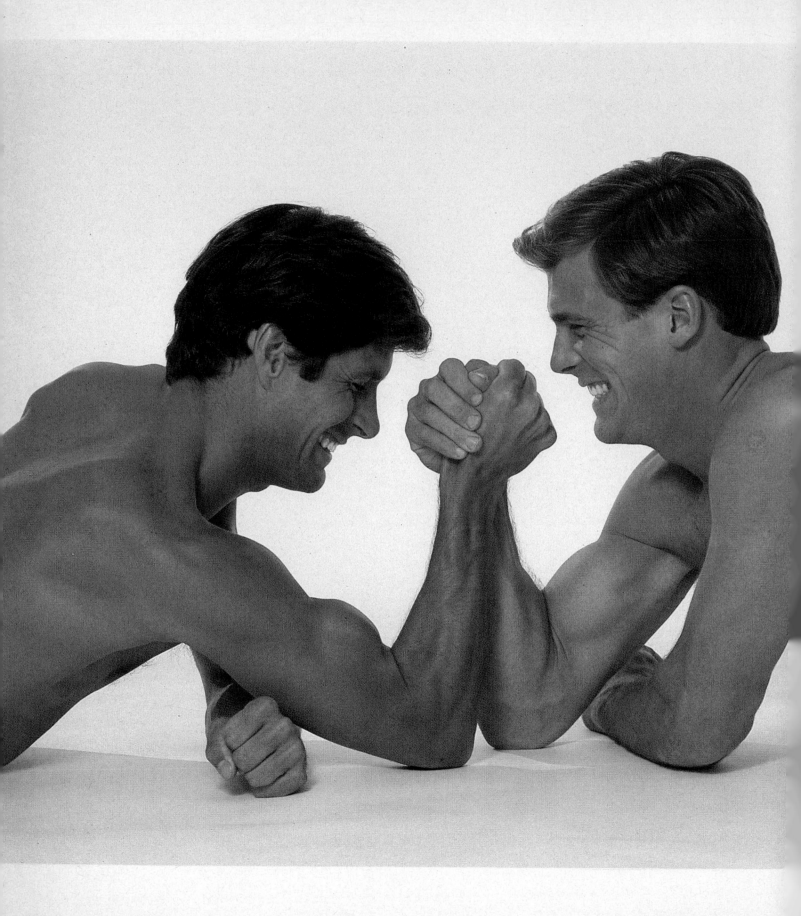

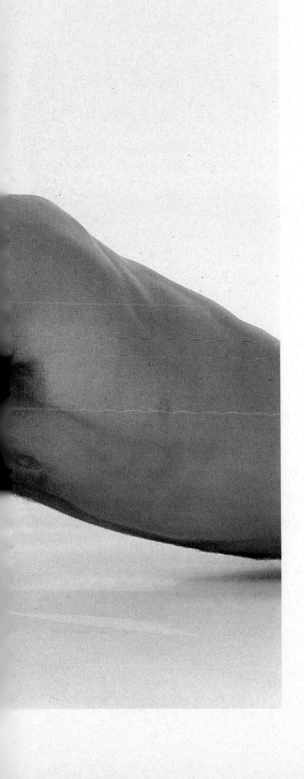

were looking for: isokinetic exercise. Isokinetics are based on the same principle as most body-tuning exercises, that fitness comes from exerting muscles against resistance. In most solo exercise routines, resistance comes from body weight (as in regular push-ups, sit-ups or leg-lifts), or from weights (as in Nautilus training). In One-on-One exercises, the isokinetic resistance comes from your partner.

Isokinetics combine the advantages of isometrics with the principles of T'ai Chi. In isometrics you try to pit two equal forces against each other so there's no movement, but a lot of exertion (for example, a good arm-wrestling match). In isokinetics, on the other hand, there is always movement. The idea isn't to prevent your partner from completing an exercise by exerting maximum resistance, it's to exert *matching resistance* throughout the exercise.

Most people don't know it, but in an exercise your strength is different at every point in the exercise. How much "push" your muscle can provide depends on the angle of the bone and the position of the muscle, both of which change constantly during an exercise. When another person is providing resistance, he or she can adjust the resistance to match your strength at that particular point in the movement.

Because they're based on the principle of matching or adjustable resistance, isokinetics are a more effective and safer way of exercising than weight-training. "Isokinetic exercise," says Dr. Bernard Gutin of Columbia University, "is what the Nautilus machines are designed to provide, but don't do nearly as well as another live person." Yet isokinetics are simple enough for anybody to master, from those who are just beginning to exercise after a long period of inactivity to people who are in good shape and are relatively coordinated. They require no special equipment, no costly classes, and no time-consuming trips to a gym.

Although it may sound complicated at first, the process of adjusting the resistance is very natural and takes place mostly on a subconscious level. All you have to do is try to keep the motion of the

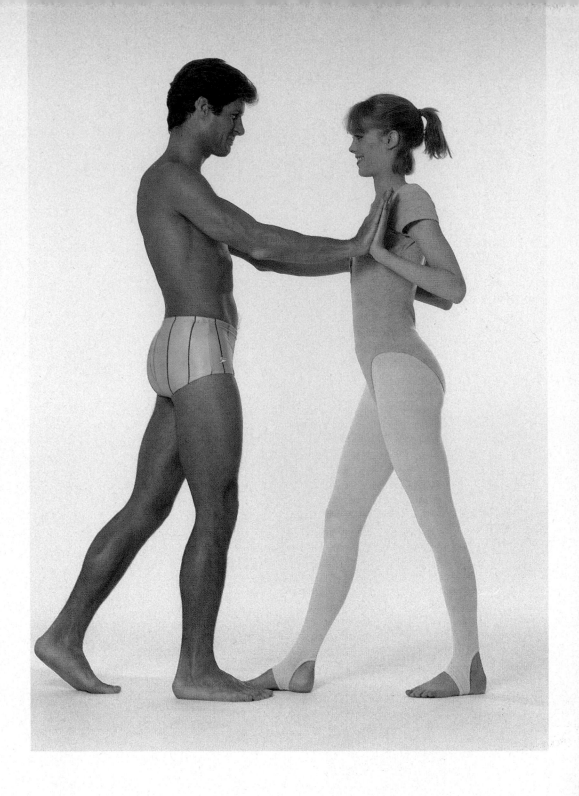

exercise smooth and even, not jerky. If you concentrate on that, your body will automatically make the necessary, minute adjustments to your partner's strength.

We like to demonstrate the principle of isokinetics with an exercise called a "push-pull," adapted from T'ai Chi. We stand facing each other, palm to palm.

First, Jeff pushes until his arms are almost straight but his elbows aren't locked. Nancy resists Jeff's pushing just hard enough to make Jeff work. Then Nancy pushes toward Jeff and Jeff resists, but not so hard that Nancy can't straighten her arms (without locking them). Each of us makes it hard, but not too hard. Then we switch again.

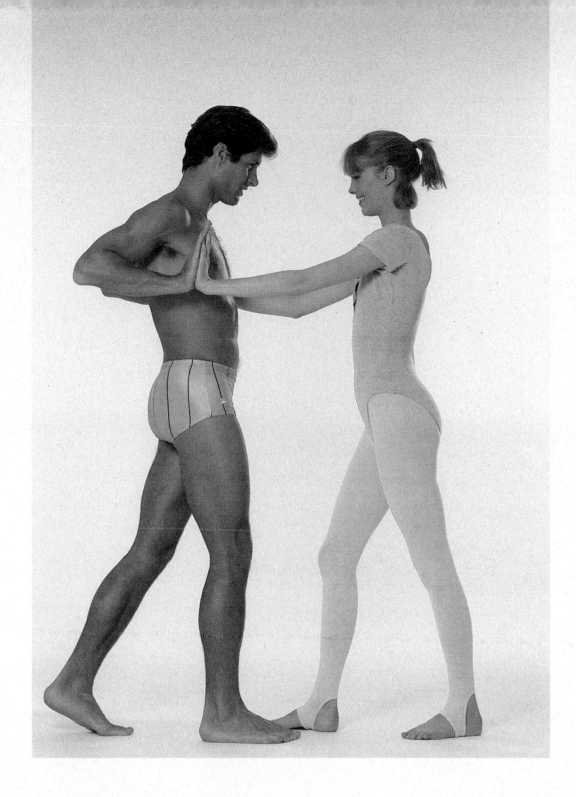

The great advantage of isokinetics is that you can vary the amount of resistance according to your partner's needs. This process of learning about your partner's body is part of the larger process of getting to know and trust each other. You'll be surprised at first how little resistance is needed. A little bit of resistance makes an exercise a lot harder, especially when you repeat it five or ten times. As your muscles become stronger, of course, your partner can apply greater resistance, or you can increase the number of repetitions, or both.

To make sure your isokinetic routine is as effective as it is enjoyable, follow these simple guidelines.
- If you're the active partner (the person who is exercising his or her muscles), don't rest

between repetitions. Don't let your muscles relax.

- If you're the active partner, when you reach the fully extended position, hold it for several seconds before returning to the starting position.

- If you're the passive partner (the person applying resistance), apply resistance *throughout* the exercise, both when your partner is moving toward the extended position, and when he or she is moving back to the starting position. In general, you should apply more resistance during the second half of the exercise (the movement from the extended position back to the starting position). But be sure to allow your partner to hold the extended position for several seconds.

- It is not necessary to change positions between the first half and second half of the exercise in order to provide resistance throughout. Think of it this way: If you're the passive partner, in the first half of the exercise, you are resisting the active partner's effort to reach the extended position. In the second half of the exercise, the active partner is resisting your effort to return to the starting position. Work to make the transition from the first half to the second half of the exercise as smooth as possible.

- In general, the movement toward the extended position should be relatively fast (about two seconds), while the movement from the extended position back to the starting position should be slower but not too slow (about four seconds).

- Stay in constant communication. Watch each other closely. Talk to each other during the exercise so you know when to press on and when to let up.

ISOKINETIC EXERCISES

When you start this exercise program, don't overexert. If you're the partner providing resistance, keep the level of resistance very low at first. Build up gradually. If your partner can't complete five repetitions of any exercise, you're applying too much resistance.

- Duration: Twenty to thirty minutes for the basic workout.
- Order: Sequences I–IV, as follows.
- Repetitions: Five to seven per exercise (each position, each partner) equals one set. Beginners, do one set; intermediate, two; advanced, three.

SEQUENCE I   *Starting Position*

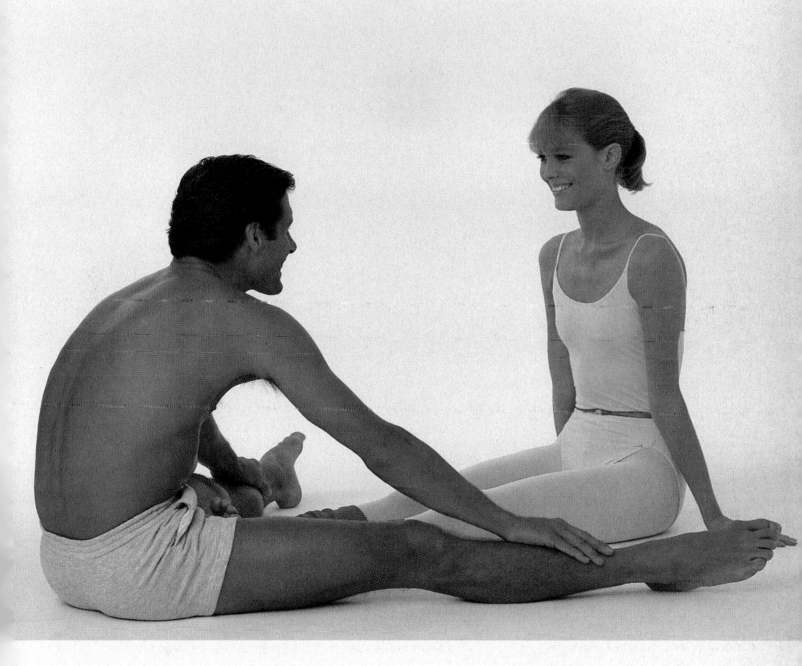

SEQUENCE I #1 legs, ankles

Remember that in all the isokinetic exercises, the active partner is the person who is being exercised, who works against resistance to build muscular strength and endurance. The passive partner is the person who applies resistance.

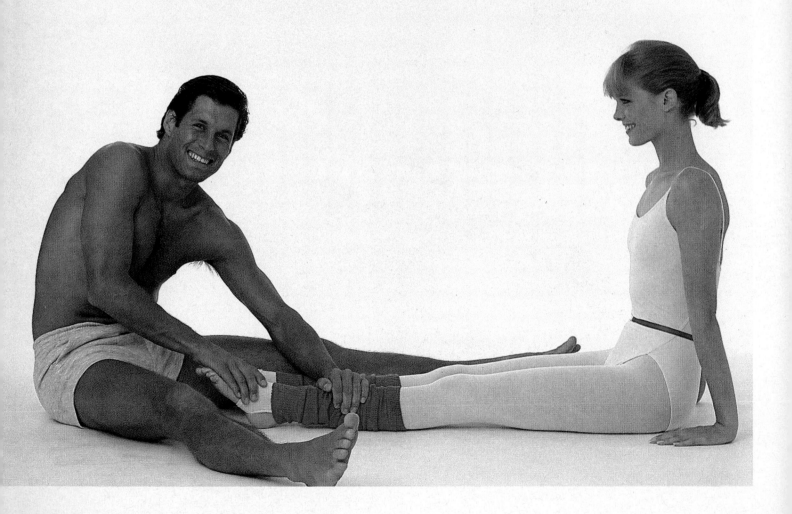

ACTIVE PARTNER:

Sit facing your partner, as shown. Work one foot at a time. When your partner is in position, point your toes down toward your partner and then up toward your head. Keep your leg straight. When the toes are extended as far as possible toward you, hold that position for a few seconds before returning against resistance to the original position. Repeat.

PASSIVE PARTNER:

Apply resistance at the top of the foot just above the toes. This may seem like an unimportant exercise, but the ankle muscles are injury-prone. Also, this is a good, enjoyable way to ease into a workout. Don't slide over it. After exercising both feet, reverse leg positions, switch roles, and repeat the exercise.

Remain in the same positions.

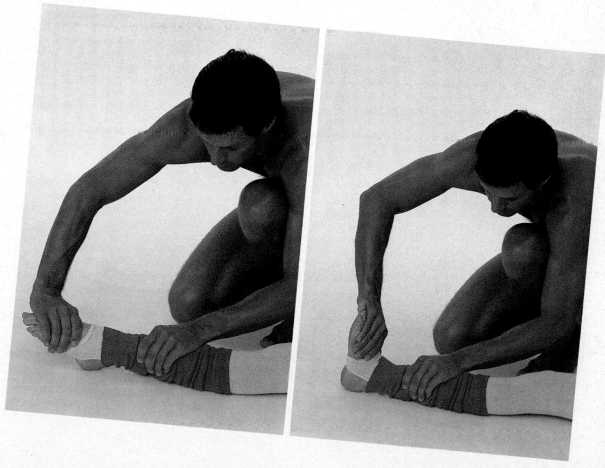

SEQUENCE I *#2 abdomen, buttocks*

ACTIVE PARTNER:

Lie back and relax. Put your arms down at your sides. Your legs should be together, your knees bent, and your feet tucked between your partner's thighs. When your partner is in place, raise your knees toward your chest. Keep your stomach tight and your lower back pressed against the floor. When your knees are drawn up as far as possible, hold that position for a few seconds before returning to the original position and repeating.

PASSIVE PARTNER:

Hold on to your partner's legs right above the knees and resist the movement as she raises and lowers her legs. Remember to apply resistance—but not too much—both on the way up and on the way down. If your partner cannot repeat the exercise at least five times, you're probably resisting too much. After repetitions, reverse leg positions, switch roles, and repeat the exercise.

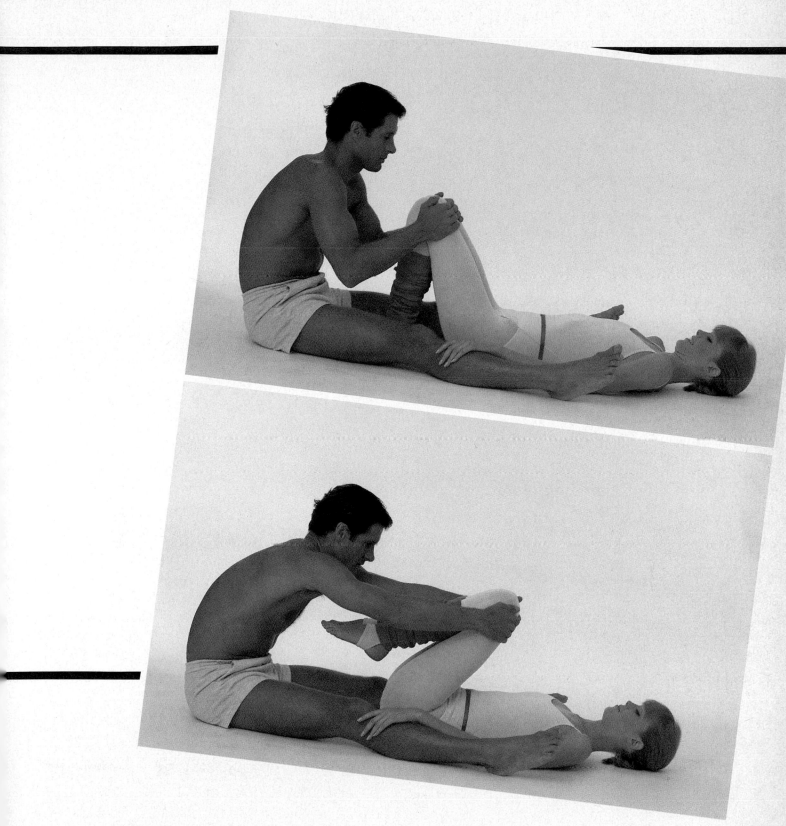

Remain in the same positions.

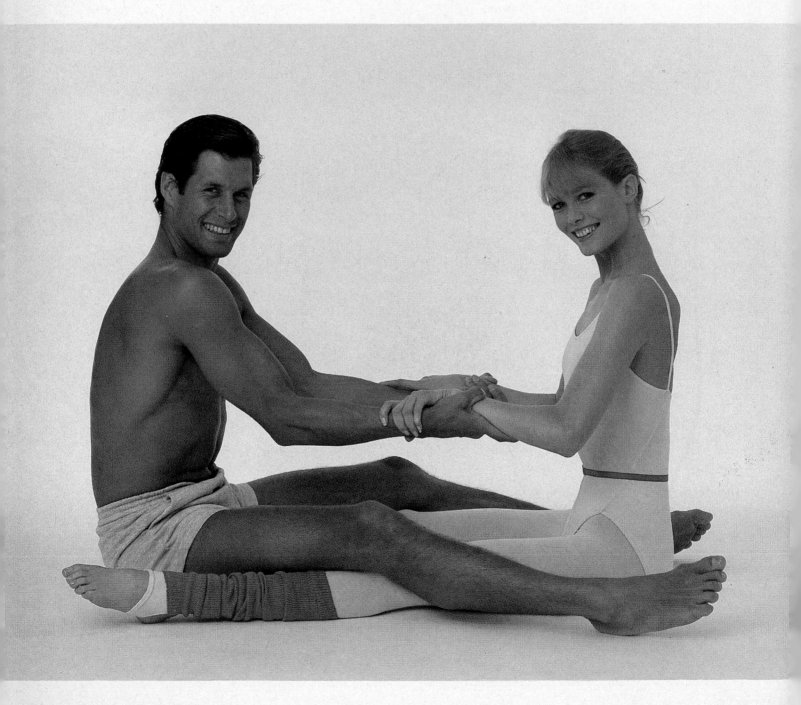

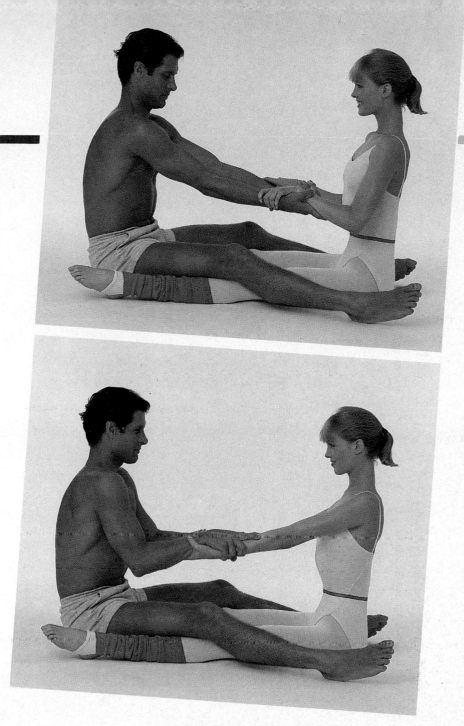

ACTIVE PARTNER:

Sit facing your partner. Grasp his or her wrists firmly, as shown.* Pull arms toward you, keeping your arms at about chest level. When your partner's arms are fully extended, reverse the motion and resist his or her effort to pull your arms closer until your arms are fully extended.

*This exercise may also be done with a strong stick that both partners grasp and pull back and forth between them.

PASSIVE PARTNER:

Resist your partner's effort to pull your hands toward his or her chest. When your arms are fully extended, pull your partner's arms toward you until they are fully extended. Continue this way through the appropriate repetitions.

Remain in the same positions.

SEQUENCE I *#4 lower back*

ACTIVE PARTNER:

You begin this exercise in a sitting position, as shown. Grasp your partner's wrists firmly. Lean back, keeping your arms straight, and raise your partner off the floor. Keep pulling until your back is against the floor. At that point, reverse the motion and resist your partner's efforts to raise you to a sitting position.

PASSIVE PARTNER:

You begin the exercise lying on your back. As your partner begins to lean back, keep your arms extended and resist his effort to raise you to a sitting position. Then reverse the motion by leaning back and raising your partner to a sitting position. Repeat.

Unless you're doing an intermediate or advanced workout, there is no need to repeat Sequence I before going on to Sequence II.

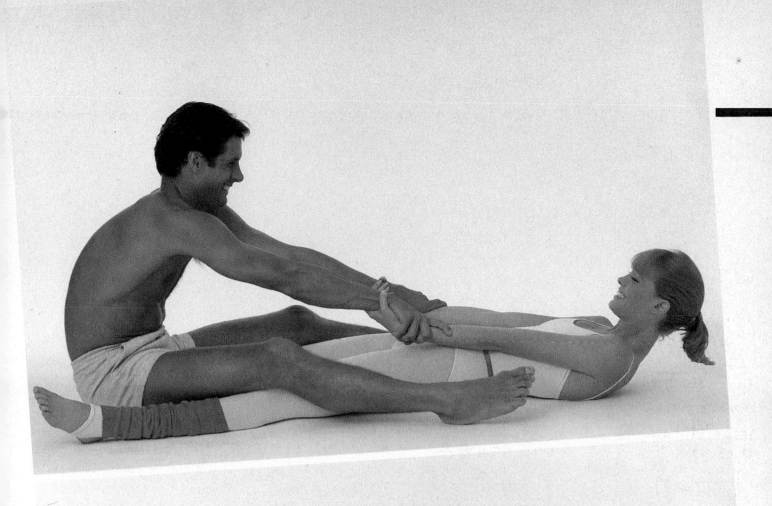

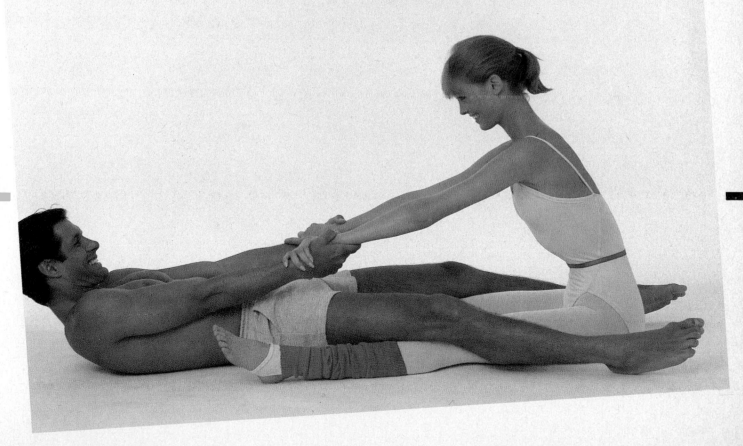

SEQUENCE II *Starting Position*

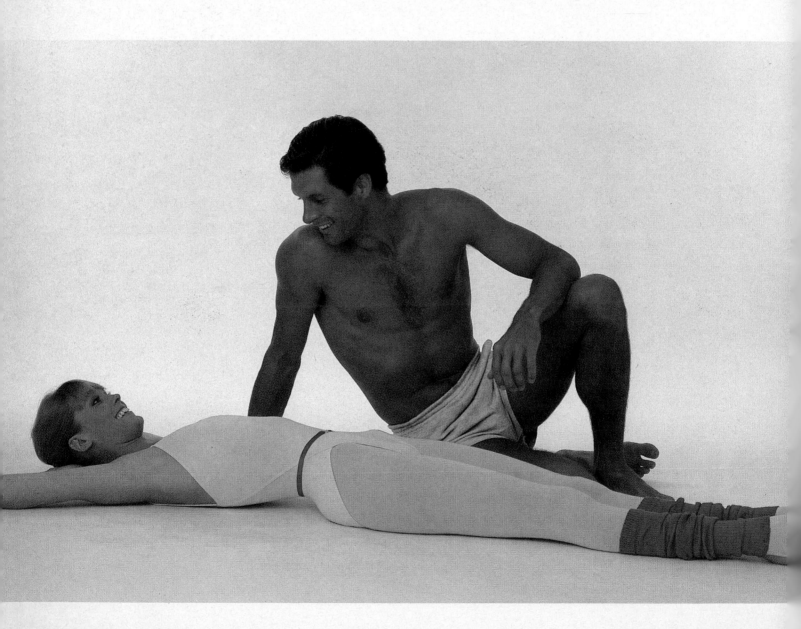

SEQUENCE II
#1 hips, buttocks

ACTIVE PARTNER:

Lie flat and relax. Your arms can be behind your head or out at your sides. When your partner is in position, raise one knee toward your chest, keeping the lower leg flat on the floor. When the knee is as high as it will go, hold that position for several seconds before bringing it down. Repeat, working with legs.

PASSIVE PARTNER:

Place one hand on the upper thigh and one just above the knee and resist the movement as your partner brings her knee toward her and then down. You may have to move forward and backward as the leg is raised and lowered. Normally, both legs can be exercised without the passive partner changing position.

Active partner, roll onto your side.

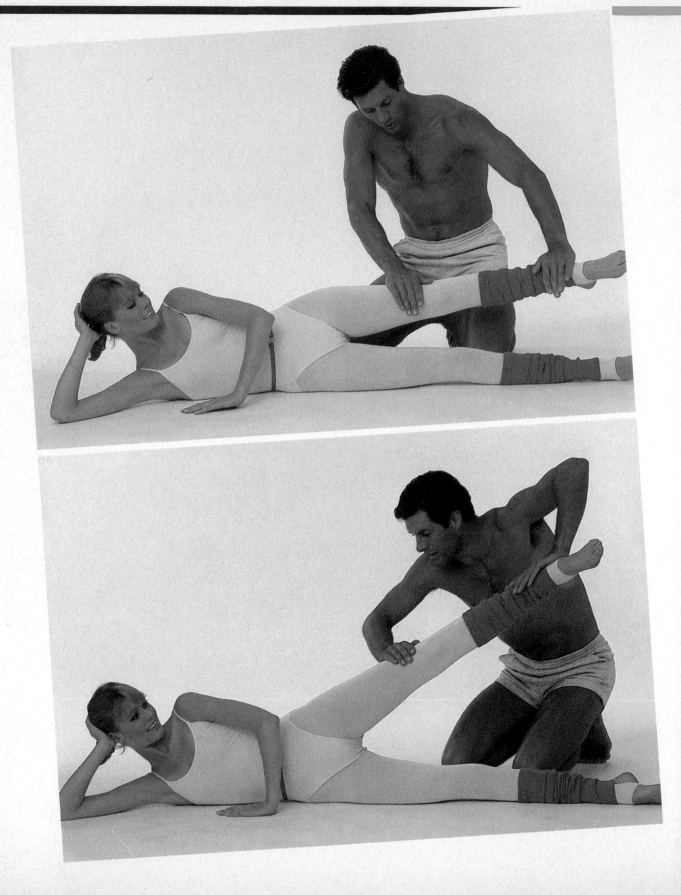

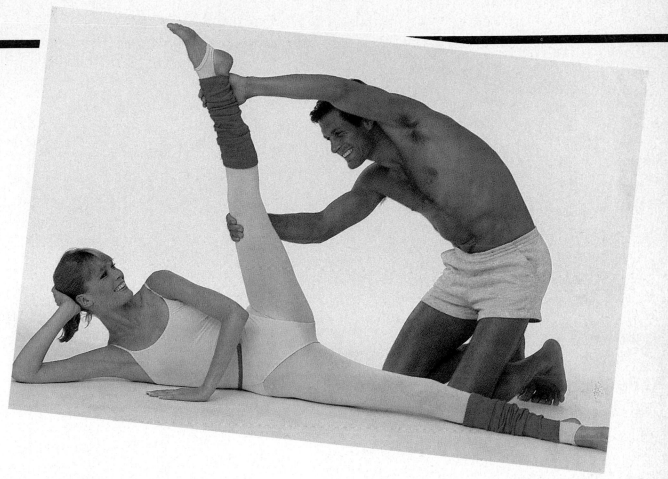

ACTIVE PARTNER:

Lie on your side with your body fully extended and straight, one leg on top of the other. Prop your head on your elbow and relax. When your partner is in place, raise the top leg as high as possible, making sure that your lower leg and upper body remain in a straight line. When your leg is fully extended, hold it for a few seconds before bringing it down slow. After one leg is exercised, roll over, face your partner, and repeat on the other leg.

PASSIVE PARTNER:

Apply resistance straight down as the leg is raised and lowered. Watch to be sure that the leg remains straight during the lift. If your partner has had knee problems, apply resistance only above the knee.

Active partner, roll onto your stomach.

SEQUENCE II *#3 hamstrings*

ACTIVE PARTNER:

Lying on your stomach, prop your upper body on your elbows and point your toes. Keeping your knee on the floor, raise your lower leg only. To increase the range of motion, keep your toes pointed at the floor as you bend your knee and bring the leg up. Raise the leg until it is perpendicular to the floor and hold it there for several seconds before bringing it down. Repeat, working both legs.

PASSIVE PARTNER:

Apply resistance to the heel or the back of the lower leg. For stability and leverage, you may need to place one hand on the back of your partner's thigh. Normally, both legs can be exercised without the passive partner changing position.

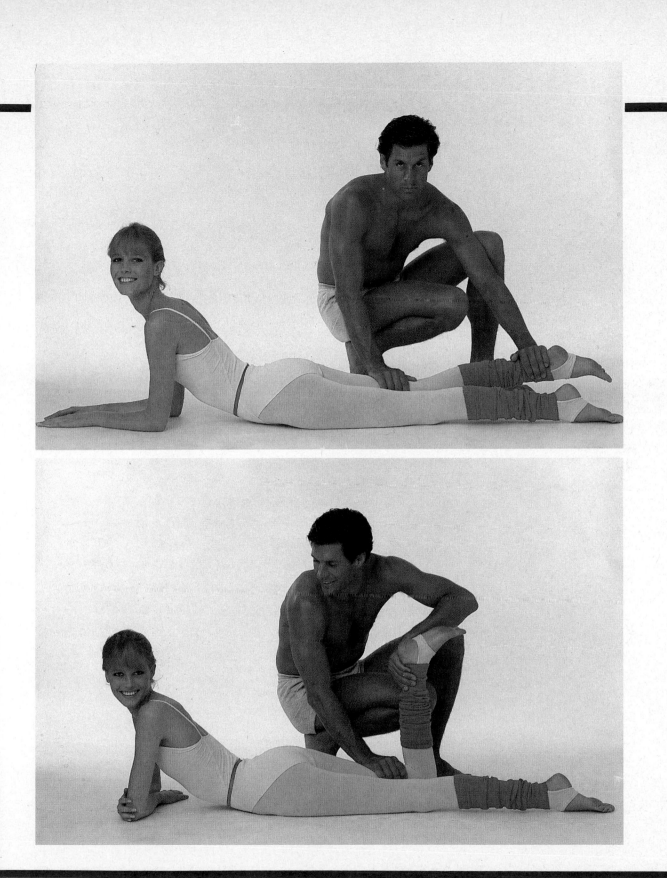

Passive partner, stand up.

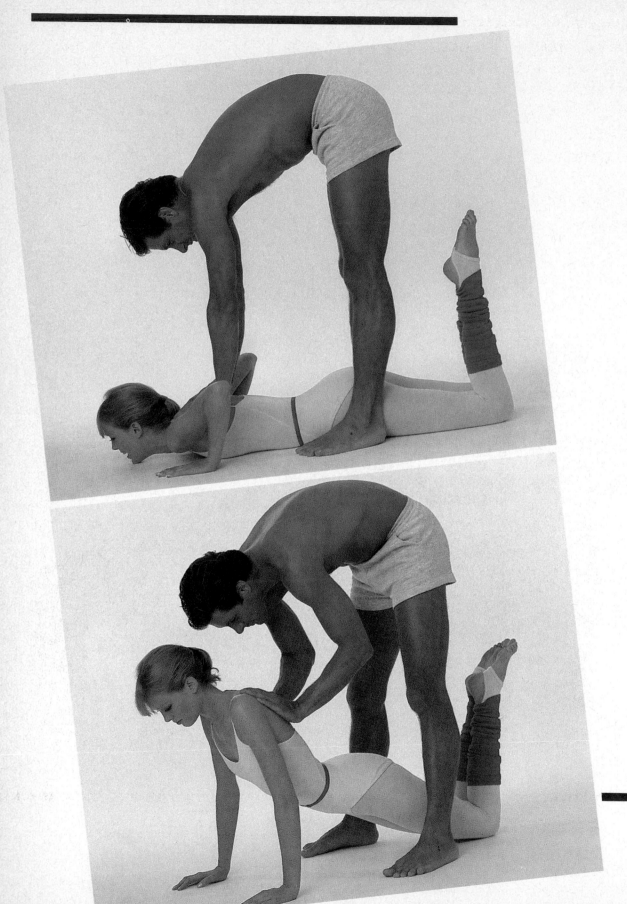

ACTIVE PARTNER:

Assume a push-up position that is appropriate to your upper body strength. Most women and some men will want to start with the hands-and-knees position shown.* There are four important things to remember: Plant your hands directly under your shoulders, keep your body straight, don't let your thighs or stomach touch the floor, and don't let your chest rest on the floor between repetitions.

PASSIVE PARTNER:

To apply resistance, straddle your partner, place both hands on his or her upper back, and press. Don't make the exercise too difficult. Adjust your pressure to your partner's upper-body strength. You may be able to supply sufficient resistance by sitting in front of your partner, facing her, and pressing down lightly on the shoulders. If your partner is very strong, you may have to climb on board and use your full body weight.

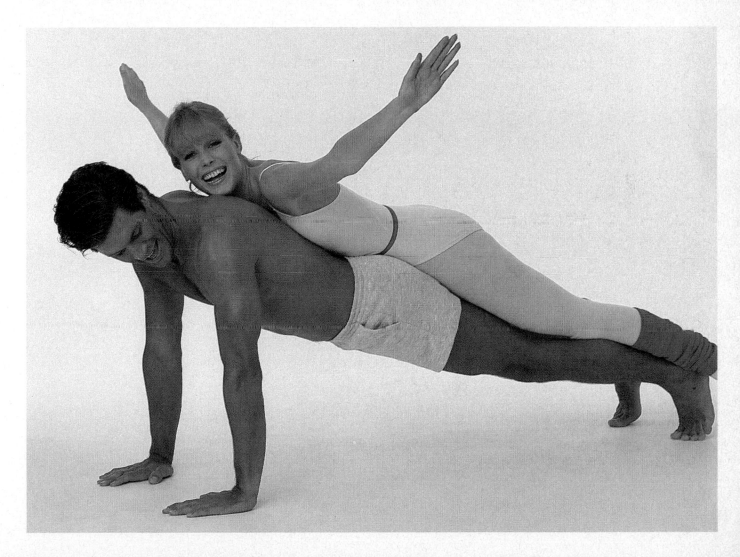

*The test is: Can you do ten push-ups in the hands-and-toes position without bowing your back and without touching your thighs or stomach to the floor? If you can't, you should assume the hands-and-knees position.

Active partner, go to your hands and knees.

SEQUENCE II *#5 neck*

ACTIVE PARTNER:

As you kneel on hands and knees, allow your head to hang loosely between your arms. Roll it from side to side and think relaxing thoughts. When the muscles are fully relaxed, tuck your chin against your chest to begin the exercise. When your partner's hand is in place, bring your head up and back as far as possible. Hold it there for a few seconds, then slowly return to the starting position. Repeat the relaxing procedure before the next repetition of the exercise.

PASSIVE PARTNER:

Your partner is very vulnerable to injury during this exercise so you should proceed with great care. As your partner raises her head, apply resistance with a hand firmly placed on the back of the head. Use two hands if necessary. Do not apply too much resistance, especially at the beginning and end of the exercise when the head is in the lowered position.

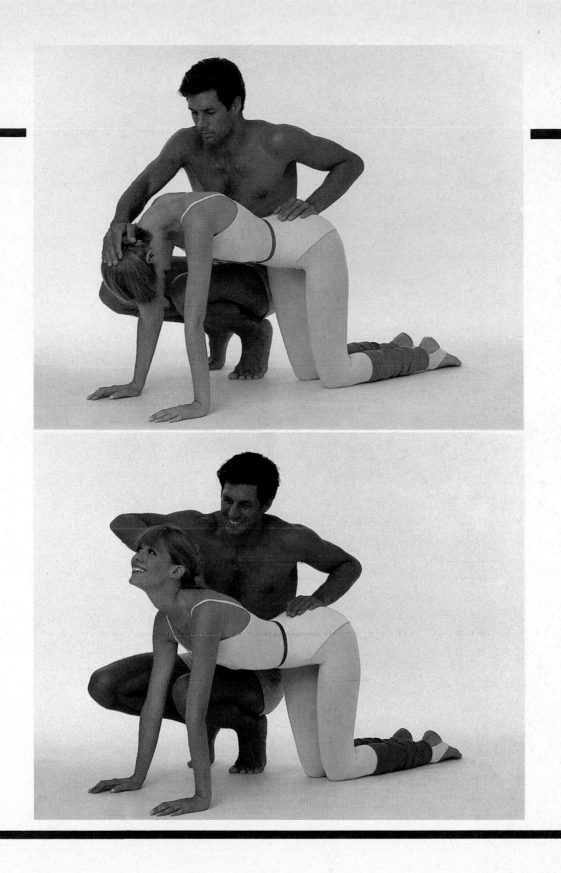

Go back to the beginning of Sequence II and switch positions.

SEQUENCE III #1 calves

Here are three ways to do calf exercises. Which one you choose will depend on how strong your calf muscles are and how heavy your partner is.* After you choose the one that's most comfortable (or make up one of your own) follow the basic procedure.

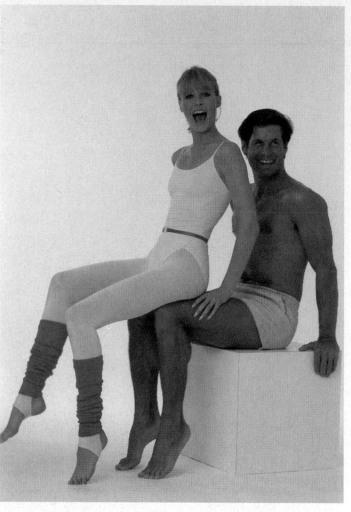

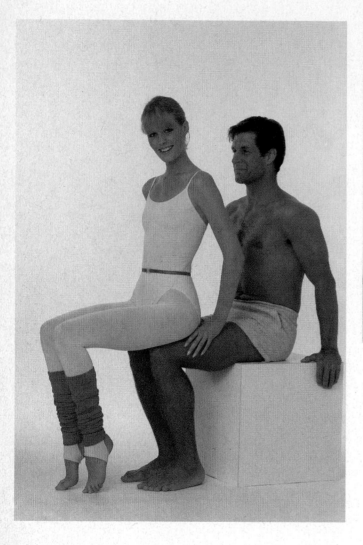

*If none of these three exercises works for you, simply have your partner stand behind you and press down on your shoulders while you stand on your toes.

ACTIVE PARTNER:

Whether you're standing or sitting (as shown) shift your weight to your toes. Elevate your heels as high as possible, hold that position for several seconds, then bring your heels slowly back to the floor. You can increase the range of motion by placing your toes on a book.

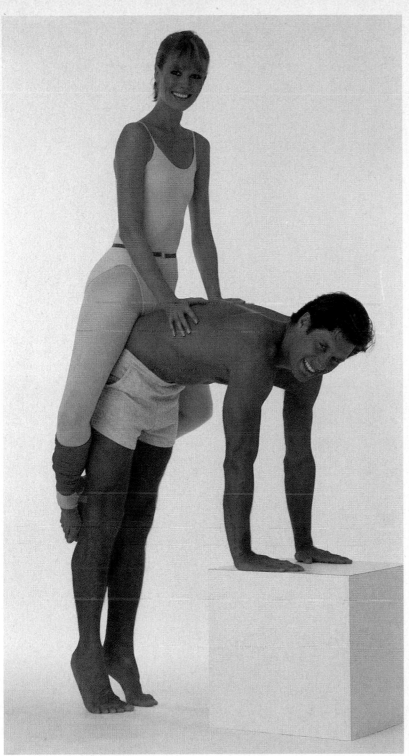

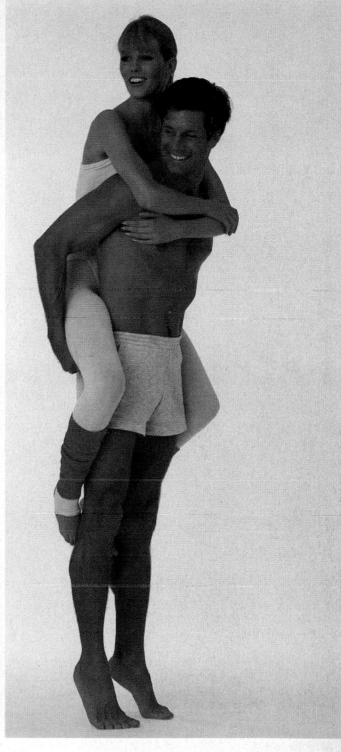

PASSIVE PARTNER:

Sit on your partner's knees, ride your partner's backside, or cling to your partner's shoulders. Whichever position you assume, remain still to avoid lateral pressure on muscles and joints or loss of balance.

This is the only exercise in Sequence III. Switch positions and repeat.

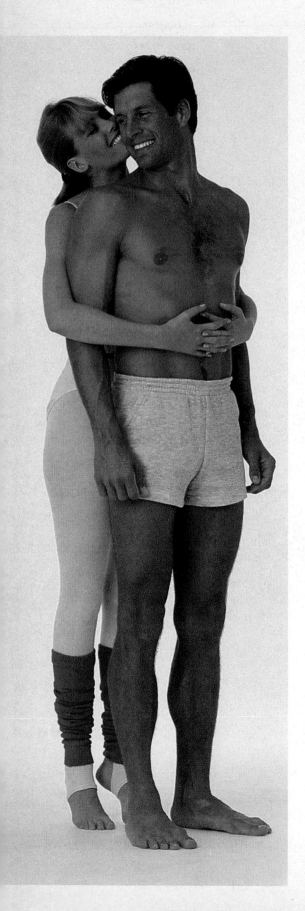

ACTIVE PARTNER:

Begin with your arms at your sides, palms toward your legs. When your partner's hands are in place, raise your arms straight out and up from your sides. Keep your palms down and don't bend your elbows. Raise your arms until they're just above your head, hold them there for a few seconds, then bring them down. Repeat.

PASSIVE PARTNER:

Apply the resistance at the wrists. Keep the pressure as even as possible throughout the movement, both up and down. If your partner is too tall for you to apply effective resistance throughout, have him do the exercise in a kneeling position.

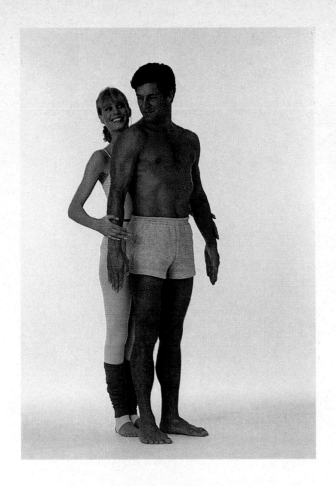

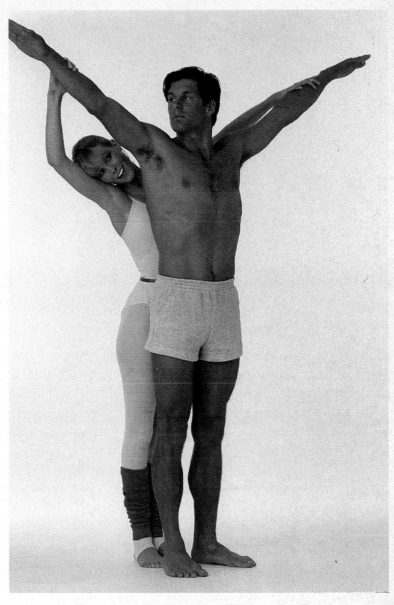

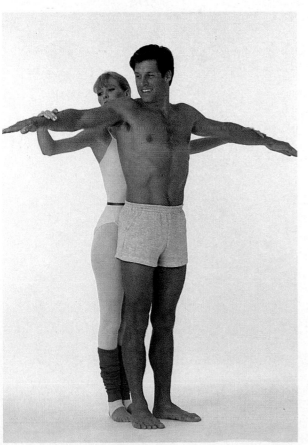

Remain in the same positions.

SEQUENCE IV #2 arms, upper back

ACTIVE PARTNER:

Bend over so that your upper body is parallel to the floor. Bend your right elbow at a ninety-degree angle, as shown, and keep it at that angle throughout the exercise. Begin by bringing your right hand up until it touches your left shoulder. Now swing your right arm back and out, keeping your elbow bent. Don't twist your body as you bring the arm up. At the height of the movement, hold your position for several seconds before bringing your arm down and touching the opposite shoulder again. After your repetitions, switch to the left arm.

PASSIVE PARTNER:

Grab your partner around the middle and bend over slightly behind and to the right.* Your chest should be against his back. Apply resistance to the right arm by placing one hand on the upper arm just above the elbow. Make sure that your partner's upper body stays parallel to the floor and does not twist at the height of the movement. After the repetitions, move to the other side.

*If the active partner has significantly more upper-body strength than the passive partner, the passive partner should move farther to the outside to increase the leverage on the arm being exercised.

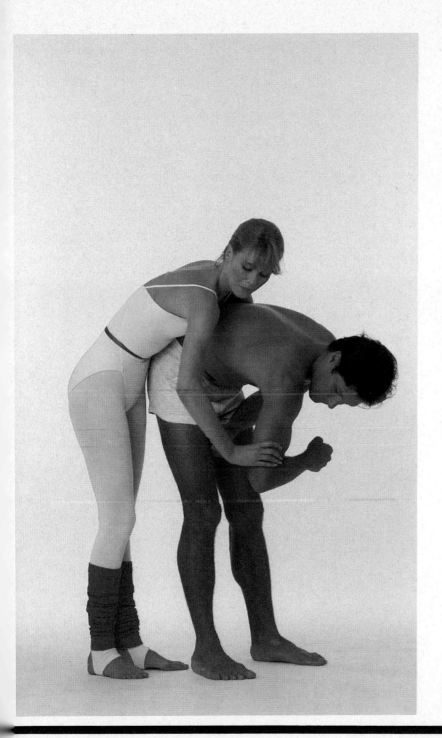

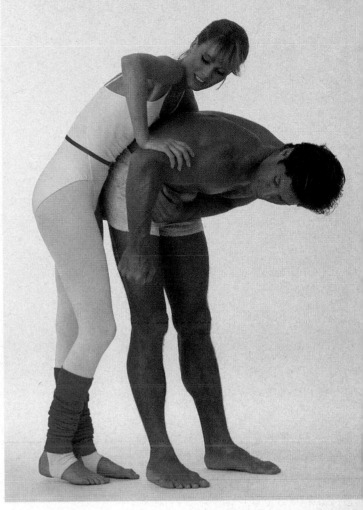

Active partner, lie on your back. Passive partner, go to your knees at your partner's head.

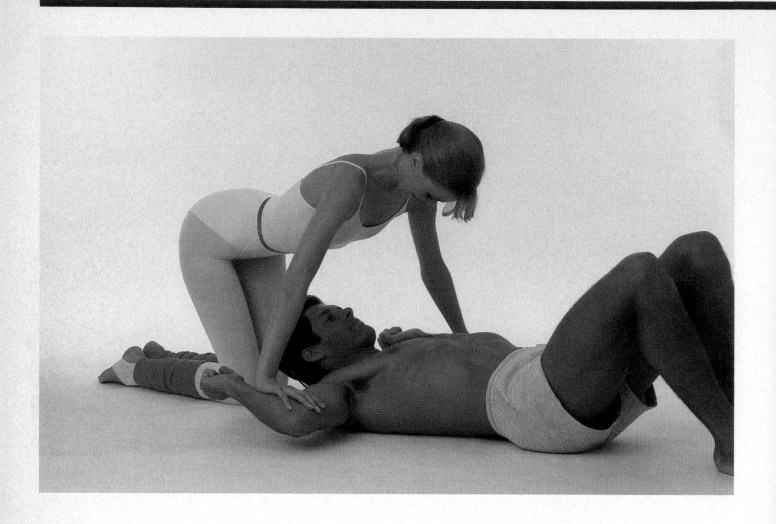

ACTIVE PARTNER:

Lie on your back and extend your arms out on the floor, elbows bent at a ninety-degree angle. Your forearms should be parallel to your body, palms up. When your partner is in place, bring your arms up by raising your elbows toward each other. It's not necessary for the elbows to touch over your chest, but be sure to maintain that ninety-degree angle throughout the exercise. Repeat.

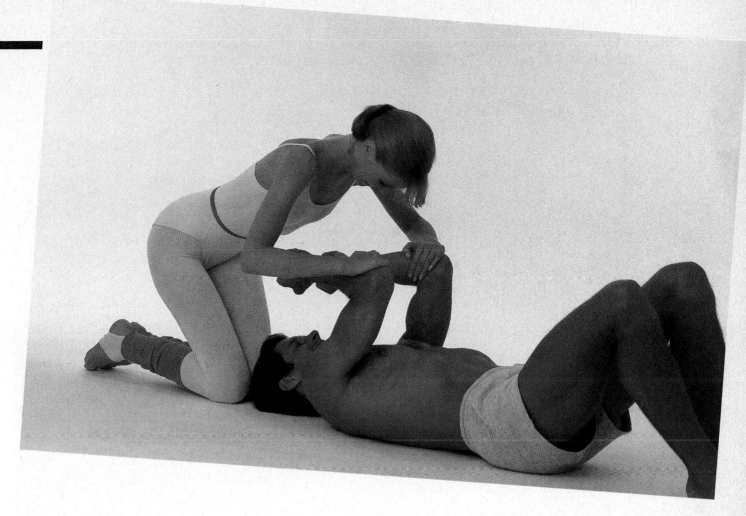

PASSIVE PARTNER:

Apply resistance on the inside of the elbows or upper arms just above the elbows. If you can't apply enough resistance when both arms are exercised together, have your partner do only one arm at a time.

Remain in the same positions.

SEQUENCE IV *#4 abdomen*

There are a variety of ways to do a sit-up, all of
which are extremely good for the stomach muscles.
Here are two: In the first, the active partner is likely
to be a man; in the second, the active partner is
likely to be a woman.

Variation A

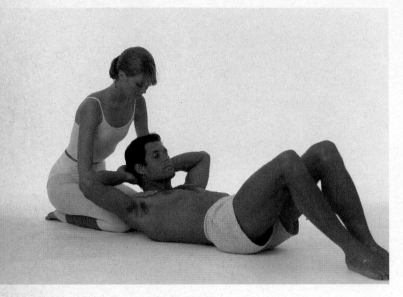

ACTIVE PARTNER:

*Lie on the floor face up with your knees bent
and feet together, as shown. You can lock
your hands behind your head, or, to make
the exercise easier, you can cross your arms
over your chest. A sit-up can also be made
easier—but less effective—if you secure your
feet with a weight or under a piece of
furniture. Once you begin the sit-up, raise
your upper body one or two feet off the
floor. (It's not necessary to come up to a
sitting position.) Don't lower your shoulders
all the way to the floor again until you've
finished all the repetitions.*

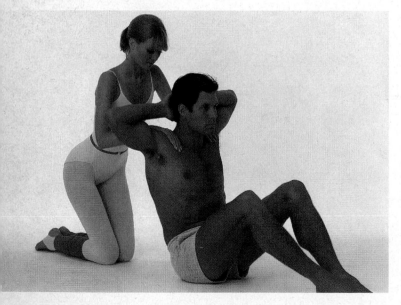

PASSIVE PARTNER:

*Apply resistance by placing your hands on
the front of your partner's shoulders and
pressing downward. Ease off when your
partner returns toward the starting position
so he can resist the temptation to rest on
the floor between repetitions.*

Variation B

ACTIVE PARTNER:

Sit on your partner's raised knees, facing him, and make yourself as comfortable as possible. Place your feet securely under your partner's shoulders. Lock your hands behind your head or cross them over your chest. Lean as far back as possible without losing your balance. Your abdominal muscles should tighten. Now pull yourself up to a sitting position. It's not necessary to go any farther. Lean back and repeat.

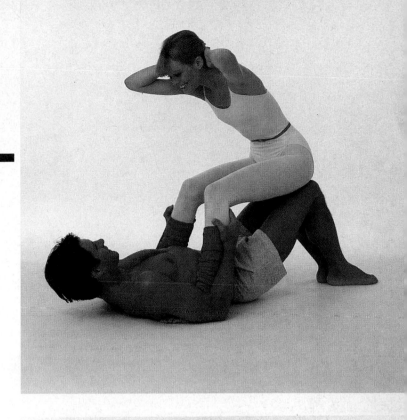

PASSIVE PARTNER:

Once your partner is seated on your knees with his or her feet lodged securely under your shoulders, put your hands behind your partner's calves for additional support.

Sit front to back, passive partner behind, as close together as possible.

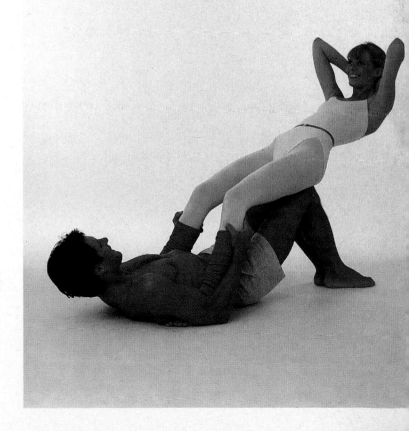

SEQUENCE IV #5 neck

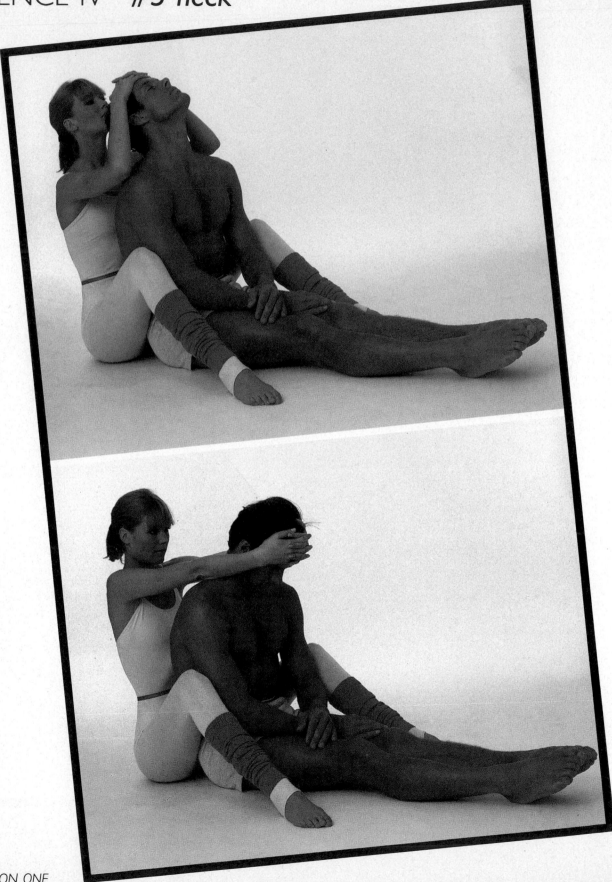

ACTIVE PARTNER:

Sit with your legs together and extended, your arms resting in front of you. With your back straight, lean your head back as far as it will go without straining. Relax. You should be staring straight up at the ceiling. When your partner's hands are in place, bring your head forward and down until your chin touches your chest, then bring it back to the starting position. Be sure to use only your neck muscles; do not pull with your shoulders or chest muscles. Like all neck exercises, this one should be done slowly and with extreme care.

PASSIVE PARTNER:

As you sit behind your partner, interlock your fingers over his forehead. Watch to make sure your partner is not tensing in the upper back or chest. Apply only the slightest resistance as the head draws to an upright position. If your partner experiences discomfort, tell your partner to let his or her head hang forward loosely while you massage the neck muscles gently.

Go back to the beginning of Sequence IV and switch positions.

SPOT EXERCISES

For people who want to work harder on certain muscle groups, we've developed additional sequences of isokinetic exercises for arms, chest, shoulders, buttocks, thighs, and hips.

SPOT EXERCISES FOR ARMS

Begin by adding to your workout additional sets of the following exercises from the isokinetic routine: I,3; II,4; IV,1; IV,2; IV,3. The following exercises can be done in addition to those in the workout, or instead of them.

SEQUENCE V *#1 rotator cuff muscles**

ACTIVE PARTNER:

Lying flat on the floor, extend your arms out to your side at a right angle to your body, then bend your elbows to a ninety-degree angle. Your forearms should be parallel with your body, palms up, as shown. When your partner is in place, rotate both hands and forearms forward without changing the angle or the position of your elbows. Keep your shoulders against the floor. Your hands should go past the straight-up position before pausing and returning to the starting position. Repeat.

PASSIVE PARTNER:

Straddle your partner at about waist level. Apply resistance to your partner's wrists throughout the exercise. If it is awkward or ineffective to exercise both arms at once, work each arm individually from a side position.

Passive partner, move to a kneeling position behind your partner's head.

*Sequence V #1 exercises the subscapularis and the teres major; Sequence V #2, the infraspinatus and teres minor. These muscles are particularly important in sports that involve intensive use of the arms: swimming, baseball, football (if you're a quarterback), or any of the racket sports.

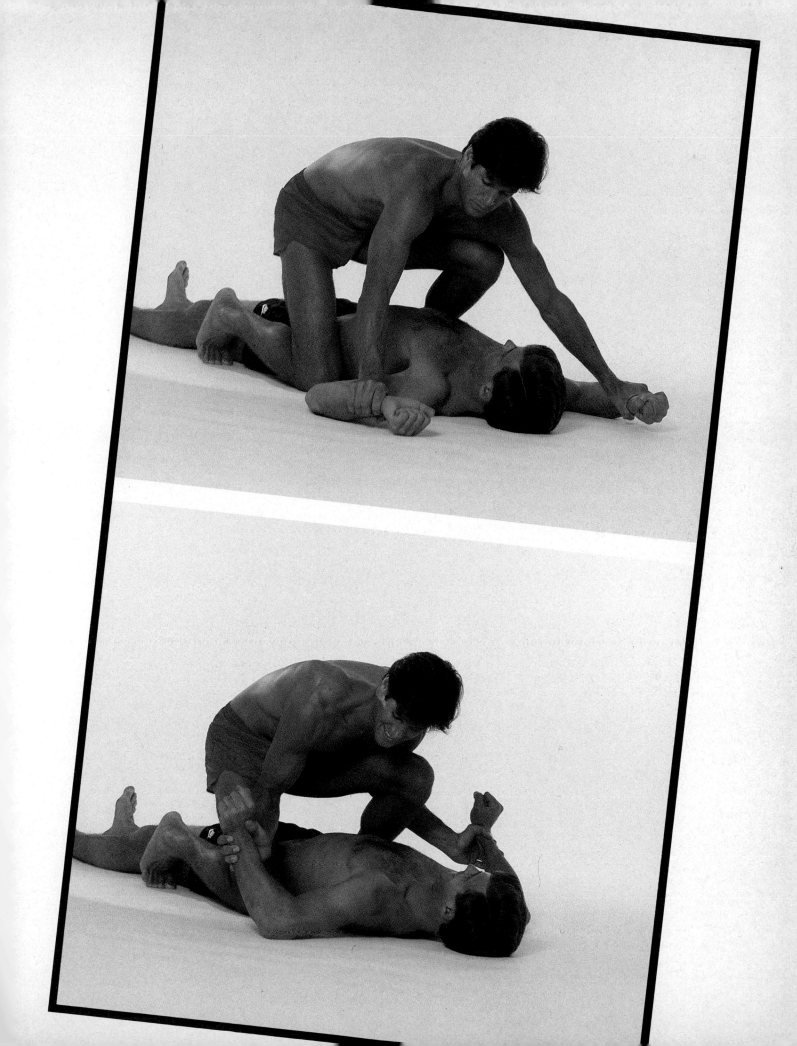

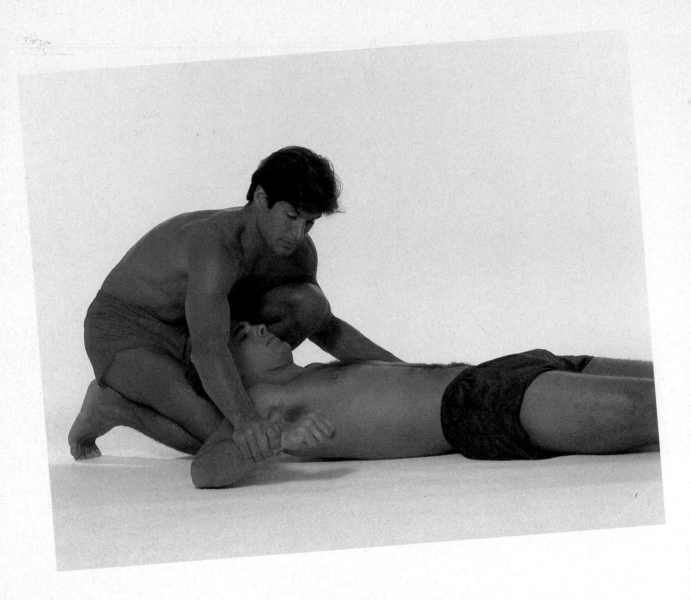

SEQUENCE V #2
rotator cuff muscles

ACTIVE PARTNER:

This is the reverse of the previous exercise. Begin the exercise with your elbows at a ninety-degree angle, your upper arms parallel to your body, palms down, as shown. Rest your head on your partner's thigh. When your partner is in place, raise your forearms without changing the angle or the position of the elbows. Go well past straight-up before pausing and returning to the down position. Repeat.

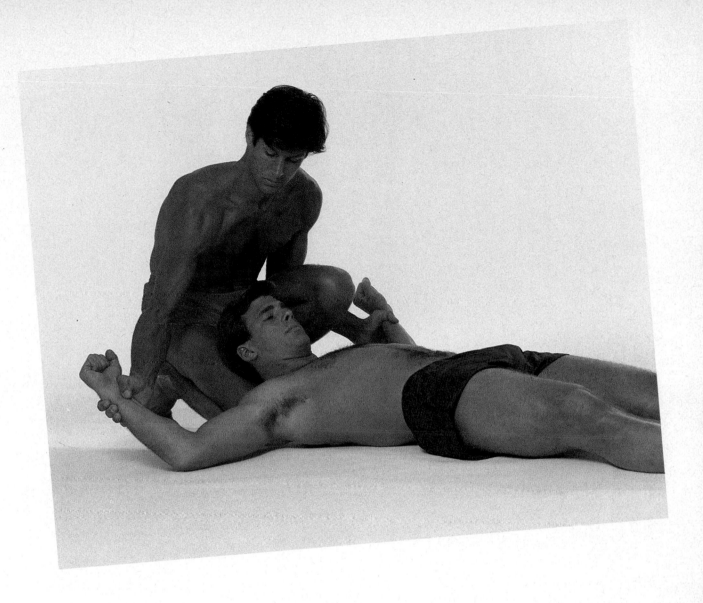

PASSIVE PARTNER:

From a seated or kneeling position above your partner's head, apply resistance on the backs of the wrists as the forearms are being raised and lowered. As in the previous exercise, if it is awkward or ineffective to apply resistance to both arms at once, work each arm individually from above and beside your partner.

Active partner, sit up.

SEQUENCE V *#3 triceps*

ACTIVE PARTNER:

From a seated position, extend your arms straight up over your head and interlock your fingers. Bend your elbows and bring your hands down behind your head. You can brace your upper body against your partner's knee. When your partner is in position, bring the arms up to a fully extended position overhead, keeping the hands locked together, then return to the starting position.

PASSIVE PARTNER:

From a kneeling or standing position, apply resistance to the clenched hands as your partner brings his arms up to a fully extended position. Do not allow your partner to "lock" his elbows at the height of the movement. If applying resistance in this way is awkward, have your partner hold the two ends of a towel. You can apply resistance by pulling down on the loop in the towel.

Active partner, roll over on your stomach.

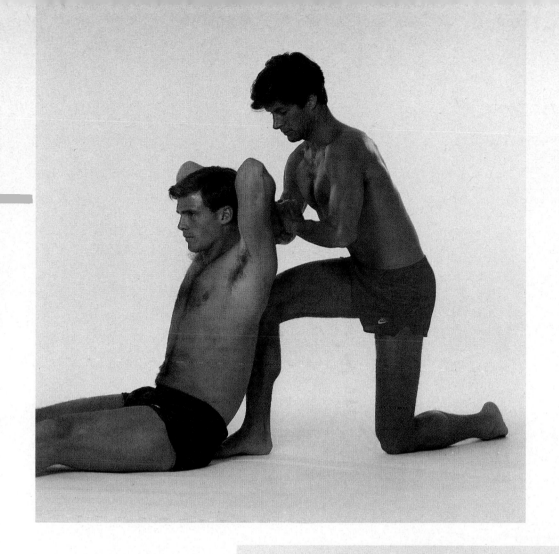

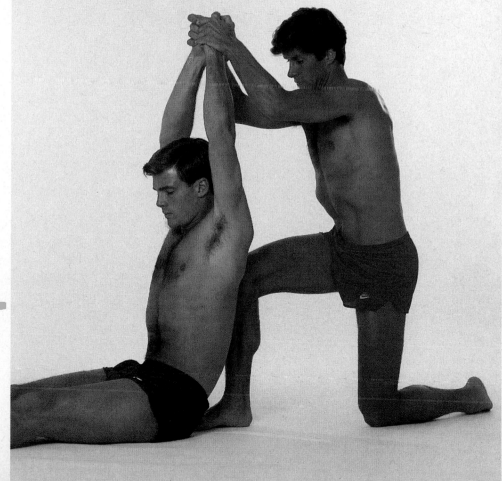

SEQUENCE V #4 biceps

ACTIVE PARTNER:

Lying face down, extend both arms out over your head and interlock your fingers, as shown. When your partner is in position, bend your elbows and bring your hands to a position just behind your neck, then return to the starting position. Your forehead should touch the floor throughout the exercise.

PASSIVE PARTNER:

Apply resistance to the clenched hands as your partner bends his arms back. Allow your partner to hold the flexed position (hands behind the head) for a few seconds before returning to the extended position. If you're exercising on a hard floor, you may want to put a towel under your partner's elbows.

If you wish, go back to the beginning of the sequence and switch positions.

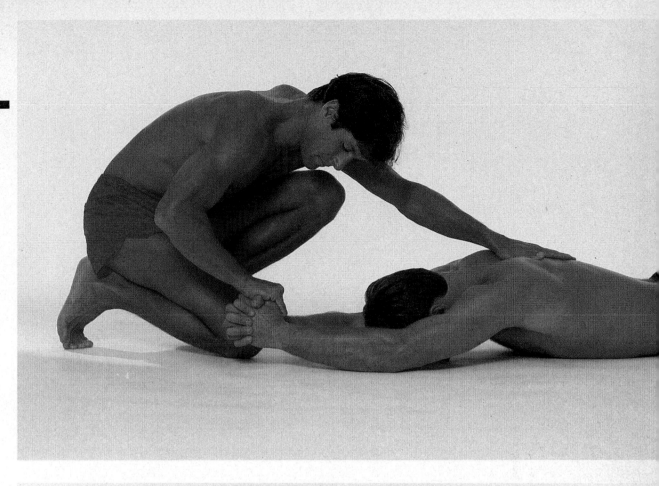

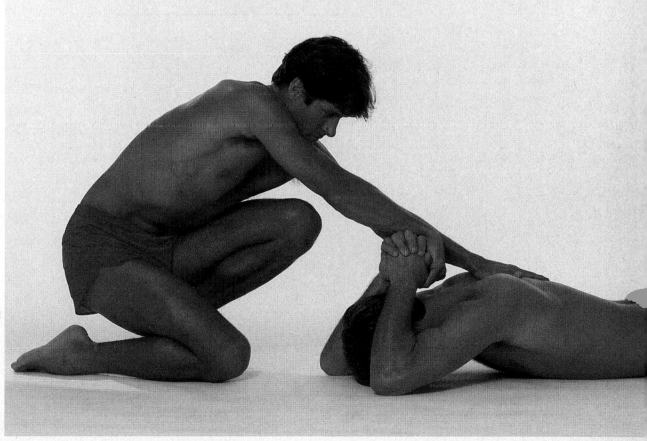

SPOT EXERCISES FOR THE CHEST AND SHOULDERS

Begin by adding to your workout additional sets of the following exercises from the isokinetic routine: I,3; II,4; IV,2; IV,3; IV,4. The following exercises can be done in addition to those in the workout, or instead of them.

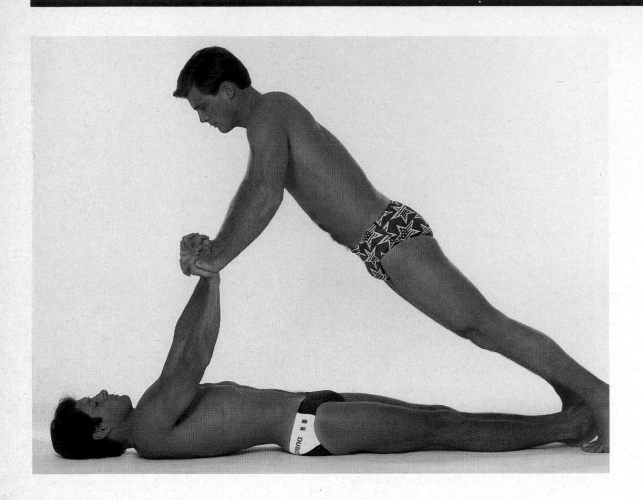

SEQUENCE VI   *#1 pectorals**

ACTIVE PARTNER:

Plant your feet on either side of your partner's feet and lean down until your hands are resting on your partner's upstretched hands. Assume a push-up position—arms and back straight. Now do a push-up. Lower your body until your chest is

even with your hands. At this point, your partner should lower you until his elbows touch the floor. You should remain motionless while your partner lowers you and raises you back to the starting position. Complete the exercise by pushing against your partner's hands and raising yourself back to your starting position. You've just accomplished a difficult maneuver known as a double push-up. Now repeat it.

*If you add this exercise to your workout, you may want to drop Sequence II,4 of the isokinetic routine.

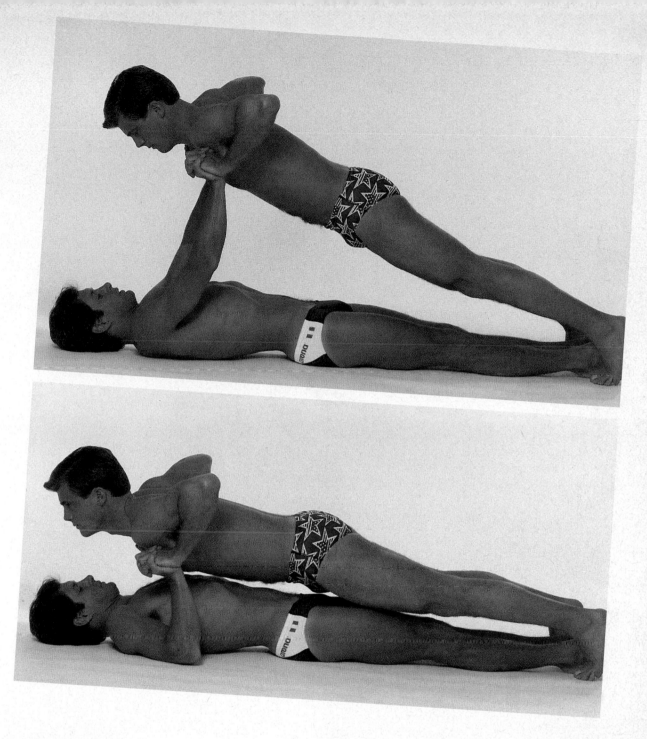

PASSIVE PARTNER:

Lie face up with your body straight and your arms extended up toward the ceiling. Your elbows should be straight but not locked. Keep your arms steady while your partner is lowering his body into position. Once your partner's chest is even with your hands, bend your elbows and slowly lower your arms, keeping your upper arms perpendicular to the floor, until your elbows just touch the floor. Without resting your arms in that position, reverse the motion and return to the starting position and hold your arms steady while your partner completes the exercise.

Active partner, stand up and straddle your partner.

SEQUENCE VI
#2 trapezius

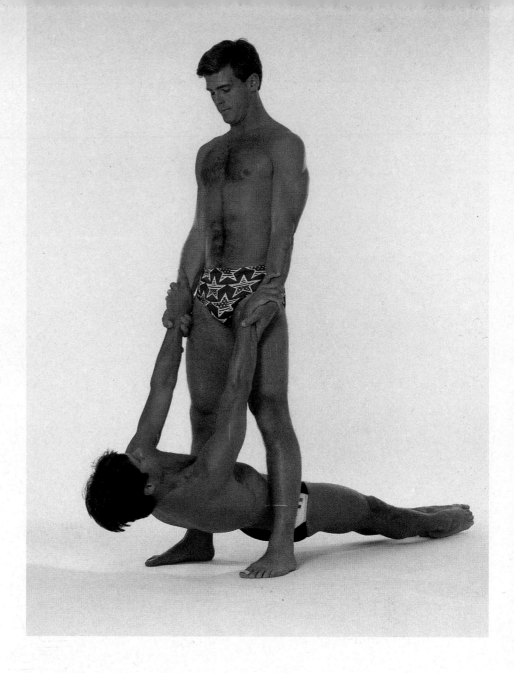

ACTIVE PARTNER:

Stand straight and grip your partner's hands. Keep your face to the front throughout. (The exercise can be made easier by using a strong stick about two feet long. Grip it overhand, your hands on the outside of your partner's.) When your partner is in position, shrug your shoulders: Bring them straight up and as close to your ears as possible. Hold that position several seconds before lowering slowly to the starting position. Repeat.

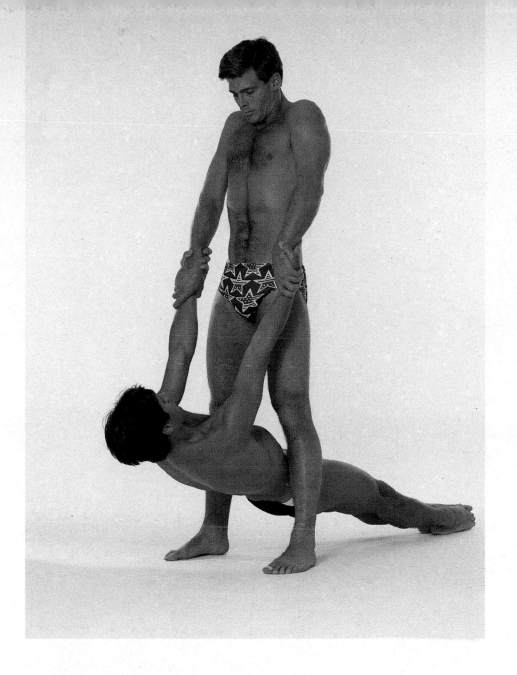

PASSIVE PARTNER:

Reach up and lock hands with your partner (or take hold of the stick, your hands just inside your partner's). When your partner begins to lift, keep your hands steady and level and your arms straight. Ideally, your body should be rigid, so that only your heels remain on the floor. If you need to lessen the resistance, however, you can bend your waist and resist only with your upper-body weight.

Go back to the beginning of sequence VI and switch positions.

SEQUENCE VII   *#1 anterior shoulder muscles*

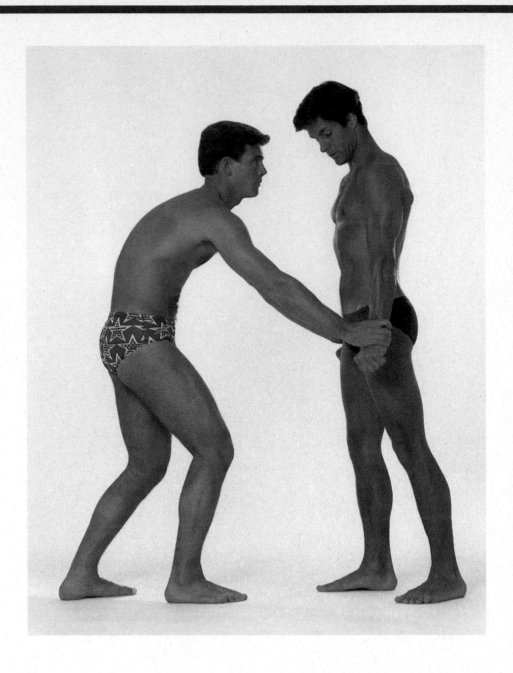

ACTIVE PARTNER:

Put one foot forward for stability. Put your arms straight down at your sides. Your palms should face backward. When your partner is in position, raise your arms forward and upward keeping your elbows straight and your palms down. Stop when your arms are about eye level, hold them there for a moment, then lower them slowly to the starting position. Repeat.

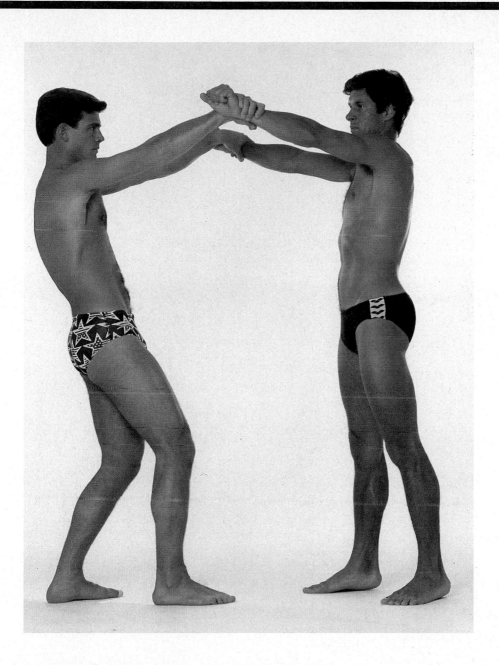

PASSIVE PARTNER:

You should also put one foot forward for stability. Apply resistance to the backs of your partner's wrists. Try to keep the pressure consistent throughout the swinging motion. To do this, you will need to readjust both the position of your hands and your body position as your partner's arms come forward and back.

Remain in the same positions.

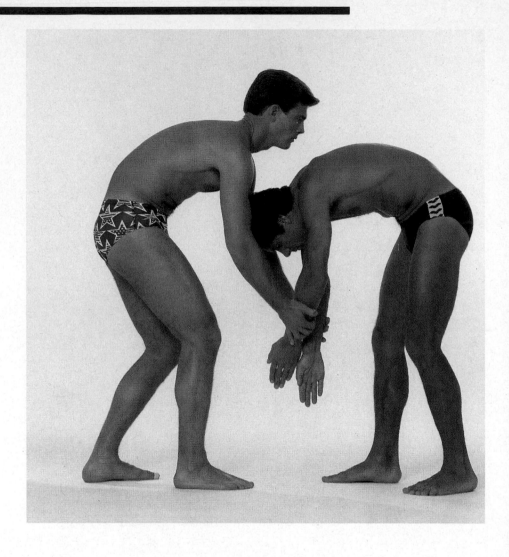

ACTIVE PARTNER:

Bend down so that your upper body is parallel to the floor. Let your arms hang down and cross at the wrists. Keep your elbows straight throughout the exercise. When your partner is in place, raise your arms straight out to the sides until your hands are slightly higher than your head. Hold this position for a few seconds before lowering your arms again to the initial position and repeating.

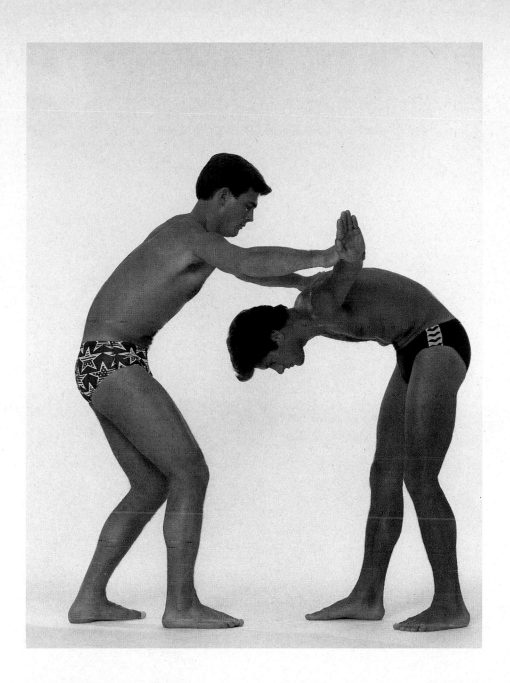

PASSIVE PARTNER:

When your partner is bent over, lean over and place your hands on the backs of your partner's wrists. Apply resistance at these points as the arms are raised and lowered. Your exact position will depend on your relative height. If your partner is considerably taller, you may have to bend over and rest your chin on his upper back, or apply resistance at the elbows instead of at the wrists.

If you wish, go back to the beginning of the sequence and switch positions.

SPOT EXERCISES FOR HIPS AND BUTTOCKS

Begin by adding to your workout additional sets of the following exercises from the isokinetic routine: II,1; II,2; II,3. The following exercises can be done in addition to those in the workout, or instead of them.

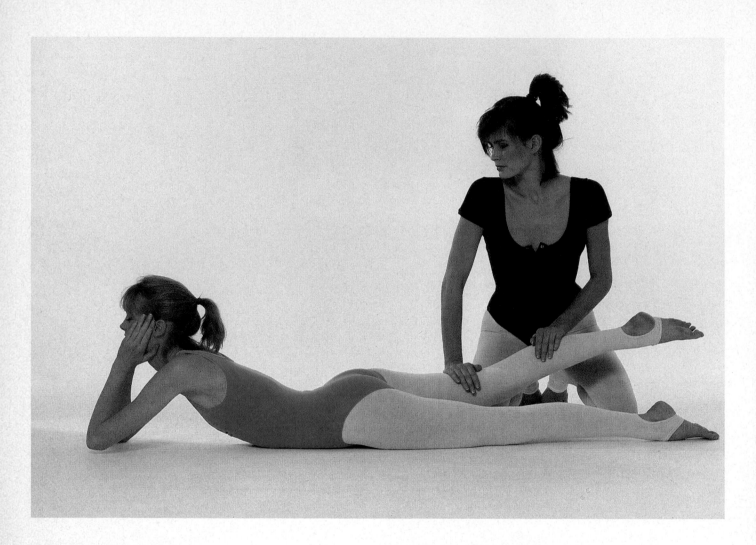

SEQUENCE VIII
#1 buttocks

ACTIVE PARTNER:

Lying face down, raise one leg backwards, bending it only at the hip, then lower it slowly to the starting position. Avoid the tendency to bend the knee slightly. It is typical for the range of motion to be limited in this exercise. Stop if you feel discomfort in your lower back. If not, repeat and then work the other leg.

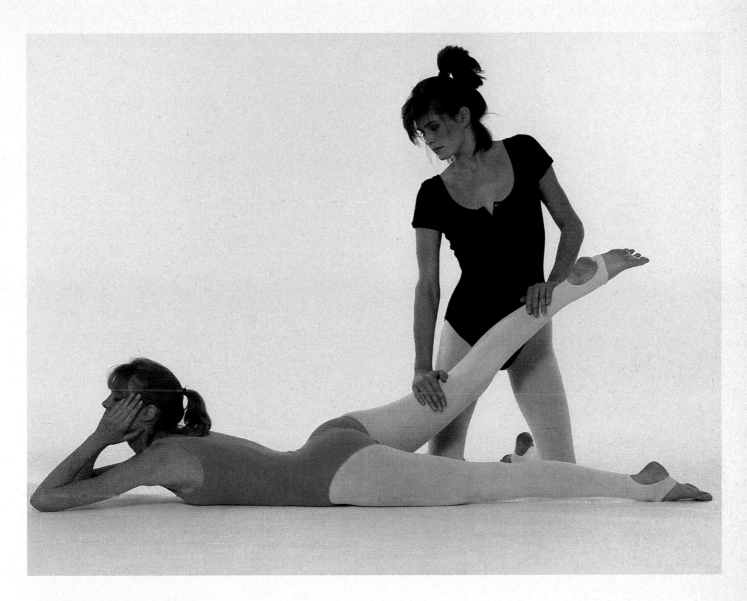

PASSIVE PARTNER:

Apply resistance to the calf and the back of the thigh. For most people, very light pressure is sufficient. Help your partner keep her knees straight by applying more resistance above the knee than below. Normally, both legs can be exercised from the same position, but switch to the other side of your partner if you have to.

Active partner, sit up and face your partner.

SEQUENCE VIII   *#2 thighs, hamstrings*

ACTIVE PARTNER:

Sit upright, back straight.* Put your hands on the floor and brace yourself as shown. Bring your knees up about halfway toward your chest, then spread them outward and downward. Your feet should be in a sole-to-sole position. Without moving your feet forward, bring your knees as close to the floor as you can without assistance. When your partner is in place, raise your knees again toward each other without moving your feet, pause at the top of the movement, then return to the down position.

PASSIVE PARTNER:

Assume a comfortable position facing your partner, kneeling, sitting, or squatting. Apply resistance to the inside of the knees as your partner brings them together. Be very careful: These are not strong muscles and a great deal of resistance is not required. The muscles are especially sensitive when the knees are in the spread position, so use only light resistance at that point.

Active partner, lie back. Passive partner, stand up.

*This exercise can also be done with the active partner lying back on the floor, arms behind her head. The sitting position, however, allows better communication between the partners.

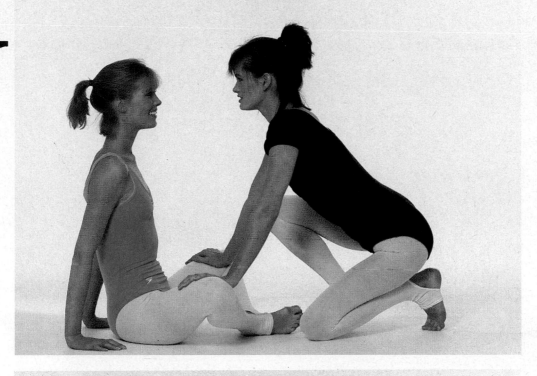

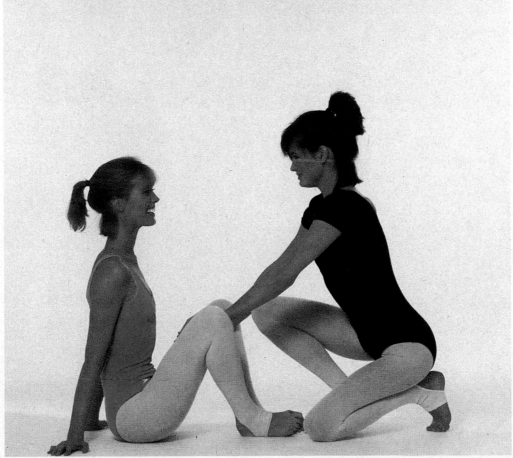

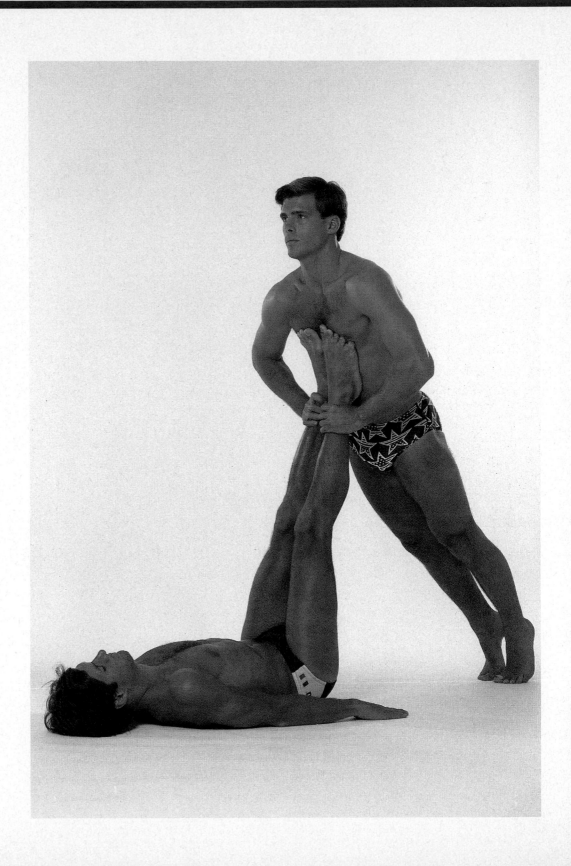

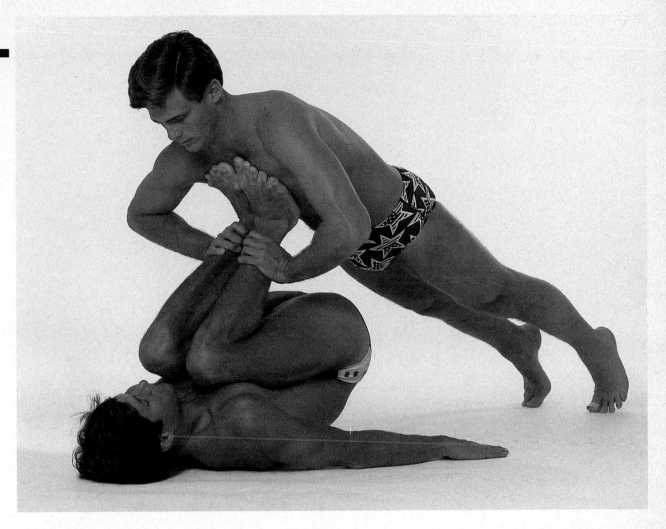

ACTIVE PARTNER:

Lie back. To give yourself a stable base, extend your arms and spread them out a little from your body, palms-down, as shown. As your partner leans toward you, raise your legs and place both feet flat against his chest.* Keep your feet level and steady at all times. Once your partner is securely balanced, lower your legs until your knees touch your chest, then return to the starting position. Repeat.

*To make the exercise easier and considerably more comfortable, a pillow or pad can be placed between the active partner's feet and the passive partner's chest.

PASSIVE PARTNER:

From your standing position, lean forward until your weight is resting on your partner's feet. This is a difficult exercise to perform, so go slowly at first. Help your partner by bracing yourself. Maintain your balance by holding on to your partner's legs as they are lowered. Keep your body rigid throughout the exercise.

Stand back to back.

SEQUENCE VIII *#4 thighs, buttocks*

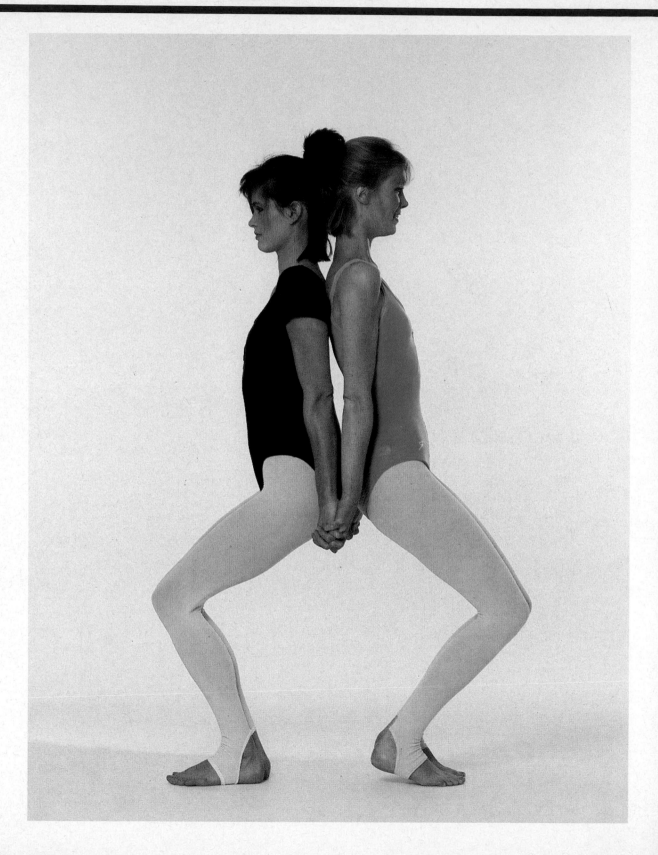

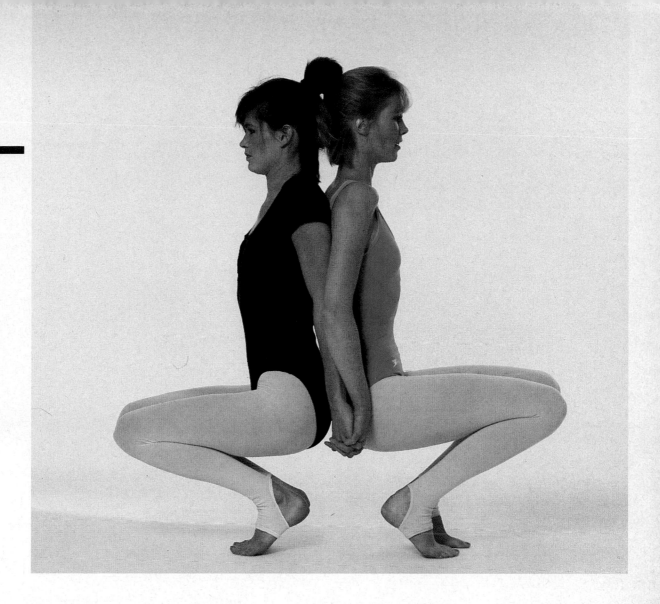

ACTIVE PARTNER:

Stand with your heels about one foot from your partner's heels. Lean back against your partner's back, keeping your back straight. You can hold hands for stability. Slowly bend your knees and lower your body straight down to a squatting position, keeping your knees together. Hold the lowered position for a few seconds before returning to the standing position.

PASSIVE PARTNER:

Lean against your partner, back-to-back, taking care that the pressure remains constant throughout the lowering and raising phases of the exercise. If it doesn't, if one of you leans harder than the other, you'll both fall over. This is especially difficult if you and your partner are of significantly different weights or sizes. The key to this exercise is to do it slowly until you have a feel for your partner.

If you wish, go back to the beginning of the sequence, switch positions, and do the first three exercises.

SPOT EXERCISES FOR THE ABDOMEN

Begin by adding to your workout additional sets of the following exercises from the isokinetic routine: I,2; I,4; IV,4. The following exercises can be done in addition to those in the workout, or instead of them.

SEQUENCE IX #1

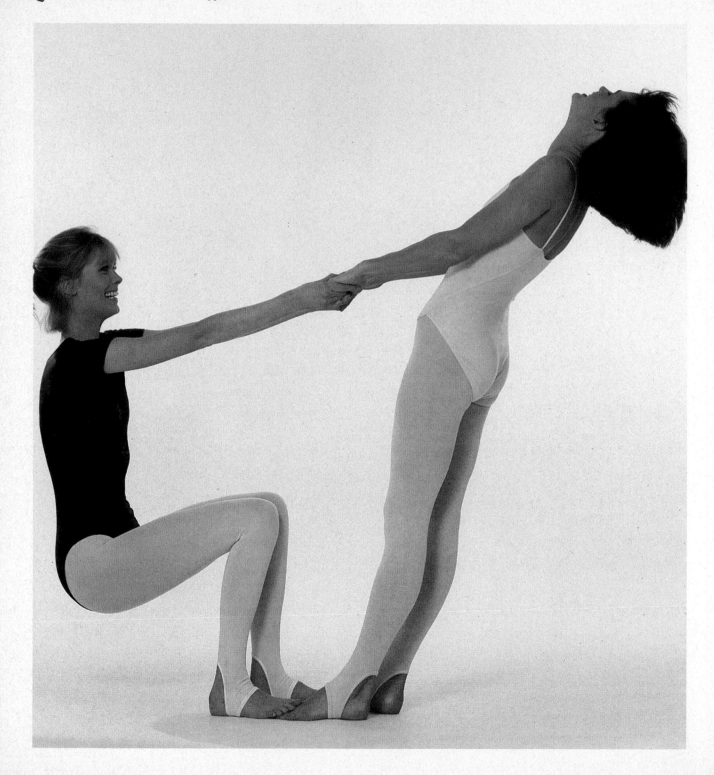

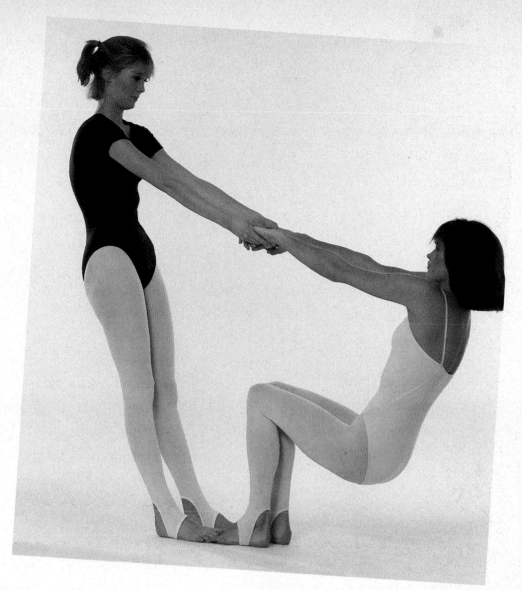

ACTIVE PARTNER:

Stand toe to toe with your partner. Grasp your partner's wrists and lean back, keeping your body rigid, as your partner takes a squatting position. As your partner comes up to a standing position from a squatting position, bend your knees and lower yourself to a squatting position, keeping your arms straight and your body leaning away from your partner. Remember to exert a constant pull through your arms. This will prevent your partner from falling over backward.

PASSIVE PARTNER:

You begin the exercise in a squatting position, arms extended and taut, hands grasping your partner's wrists, leaning backward. As your partner begins to squat, you should come up to a standing position, back and arms straight, knees locked. Your arms should remain straight throughout the exercise in order to maintain an even resistance through the raising and lowering phases of the exercise.

Face each other on your knees.

SEQUENCE IX *#2*

ACTIVE PARTNER:

Kneel knee to knee with your partner. Grasp her wrists and lean back until your arms are straight. They should remain straight throughout the exercise. When your partner is in position, lean back as far as you can, keeping your back straight and your knees together. Gradually pull your partner to an upright position. At that point, reverse the motion and resist your partner's efforts to raise you to an upright position.

PASSIVE PARTNER:

As your partner begins to lean back, keep your arms extended and resist her effort to raise you to an upright position. Then reverse the motion by leaning back and raising your partner to an upright position. Go slowly at first. If you can't lean back far enough, try grasping each other at the elbows. Repeat.

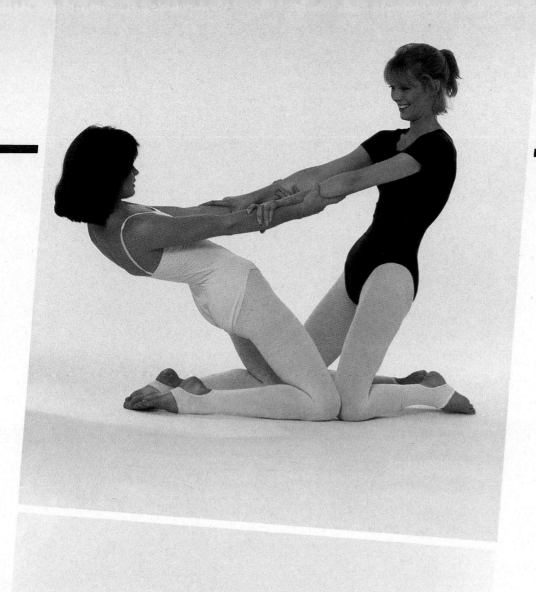

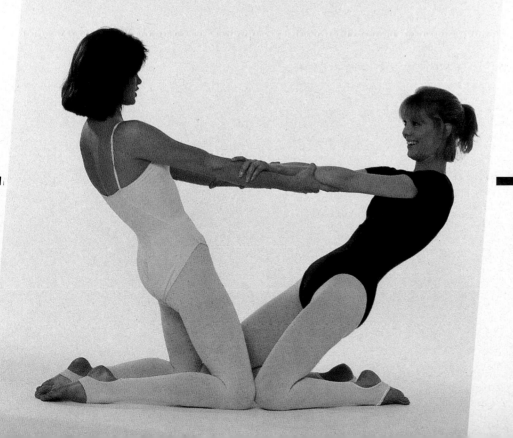

Lie on your backs, buttocks to buttocks, feet in the air.

115

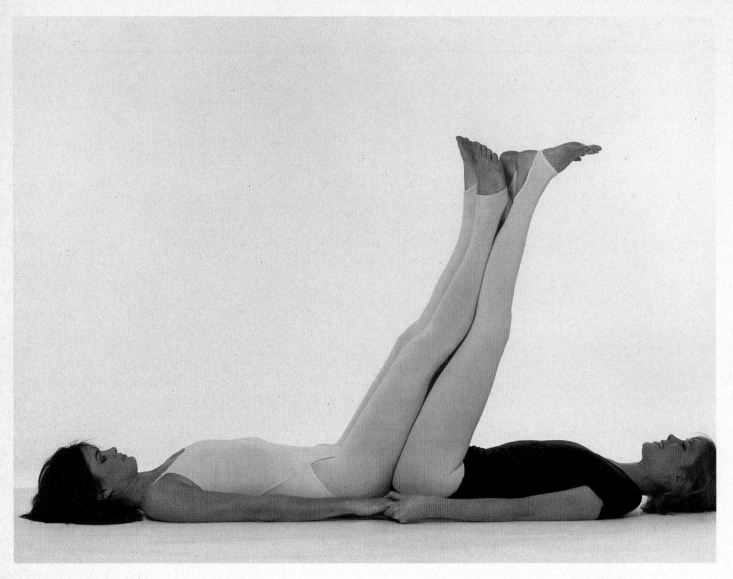

SEQUENCE IX *#3*

ACTIVE PARTNER:

Lie with your head and back flat against the floor and your legs extended at a right angle to your body, as shown. Keep your stomach tight and your legs as straight as possible throughout the exercise. You can hold your partner's hands for balance and stability. When your partner is in place, bring your legs down slowly toward your partner. Push as far as possible without bending your knees or splitting your legs. At that point, reverse the motion and resist your partner's efforts to push his or her legs toward you.

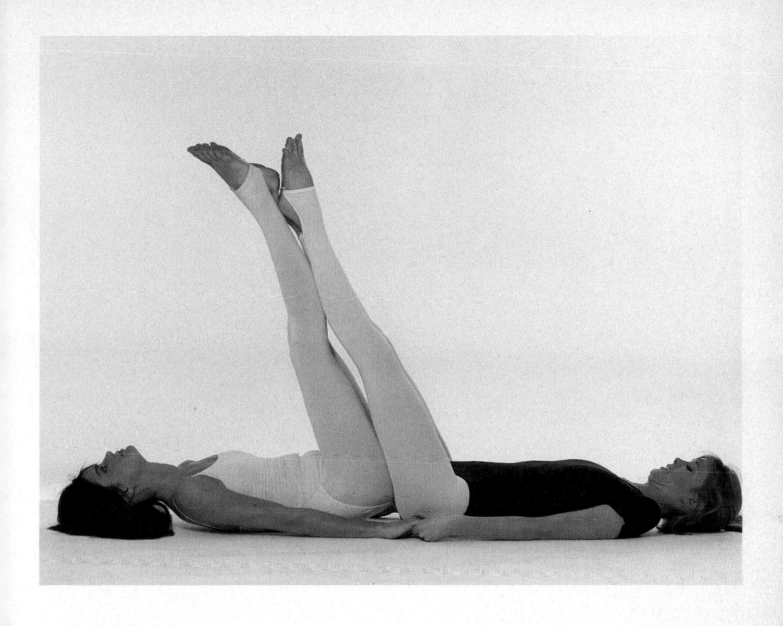

PASSIVE PARTNER:

Lie down on your back, press your buttocks tightly against your partner's buttocks, and extend your legs straight up against hers. As your partner's legs begin to push down toward you, keep your legs straight and resist the movement. Then reverse the motion by raising your legs and pushing toward your partner. Go slowly at first. Repeat.

There is no need to repeat this sequence.

STEP THREE/
Cardiovascular Endurance

AEROBICS

Your heart is like any other muscle in your body: if you don't exercise it, it atrophies; it literally gets smaller. To keep your heart strong and your blood moving, you need to get out and *do* something regularly—running, swimming, walking, cycling, dancing, skating, or whatever you need to be active.

Active exercises like these are the most important part of a well-balanced exercise routine from the point of view of general health. These aerobic exercises do the most to help you reduce the risks associated with coronary heart disease and to help you burn up hundreds of calories each time you exercise.

But for this activity to really benefit your body, it has to have sufficient intensity and duration. To satisfy the requirements of aerobic exercise, the activity you engage in must bring your heartbeat to sixty to eighty-five percent of your maximum heart rate, and it must last fifteen to thirty minutes. You can estimate your maximum heart rate by

subtracting your age from the number 220. For example, the *maximum* heart rate for a forty-year-old is 180 and the desirable heart rate range is 108 to 153; the maximum for a twenty-year-old would be 200 and the range would be 120 to 170. Beginners should exercise near sixty percent of their maximum heart rate and work up only gradually to eighty-five percent.*

Ideally, you should be able to perform these activities without undue strain. The test we use is the "Talk Test": if you're exercising at the proper intensity level, you should be able to converse with your partner without strain.

The Joys of Swimming. Although any number of sports can give your heart a good workout, some

---

*To estimate your heart rate, count your heartbeats by taking your pulse for ten seconds immediately after completing an exercise and multiplying by six. The best place to take your pulse is over the carotid artery in the neck, just under your jaw.

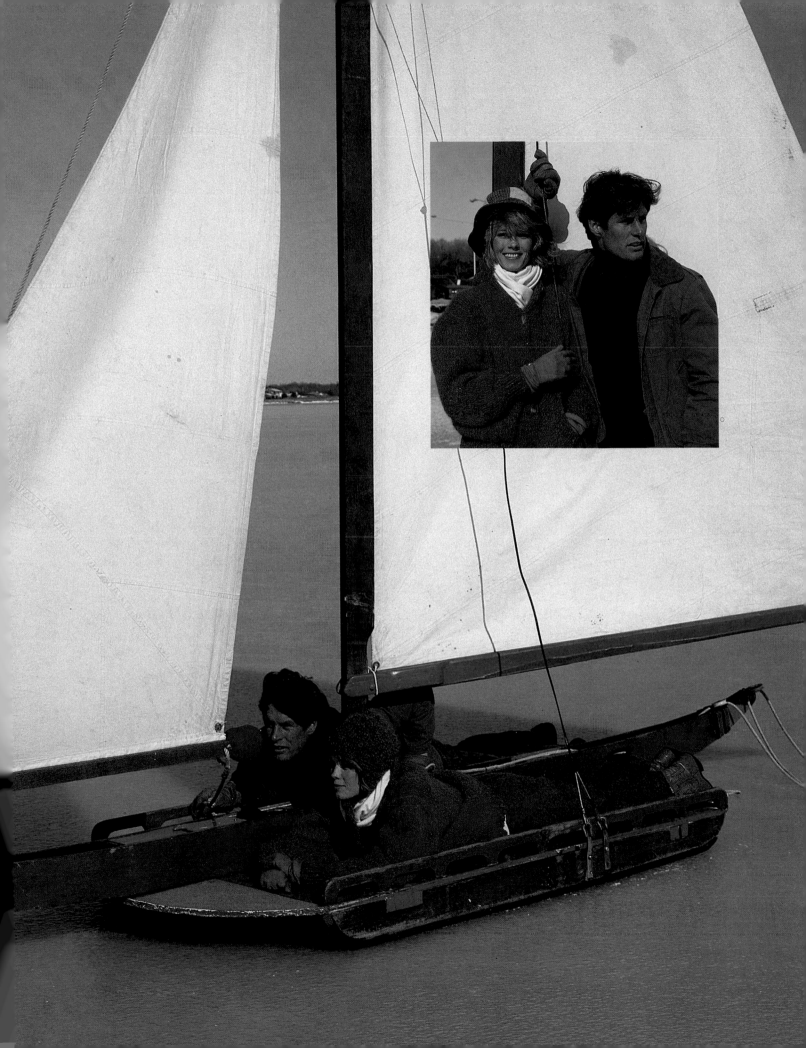

are more effective than others. We both play a variety of sports, but for cardiovascular fitness, we agree with the experts who say that swimming provides the best all-around exercise.

Dr. Albert Kattus, director of cardiac rehabilitation at Santa Monica Hospital in California, says that when you swim, "you're using your entire body, unlike jogging and cycling, which benefit the legs. In racket sports you work one side of the body more than the other." Despite the inconveniences of finding an adequate pool, more and more Americans are recognizing the advantages of swimming. According to a recent survey by Harris Polls, 26 million adults swim on a regular basis whereas only 17 million adults jog regularly.

Swimming doesn't place the same stress on your joints that most other sports do. If you're overweight, jogging can be especially hard on your ankles and knees. If you run consistently on hard surfaces, you can get shin splints or other ailments, or that added stress can travel up the body and give you severe back problems.

Although swimming is our first choice, the best approach to exercise is adaptability. You should be able to enjoy whatever kind of aerobic exercise is most readily available. We were on a shoot in Miami for three days once and the hotel pool was terrible. It was so small that a "lap" would have been three strokes and a flip turn. The only physical effect of swimming in it was dizziness. So instead of swimming, we jumped rope, then ran on the soft sand along the beach (running on sand is harder work than running on a more solid surface, so you get a better workout—and it prevents shin splints). Then we dipped into the ocean to cool off.

SPORTS FOR TWO

There are many sports that two people can play together. We break them down into three groups. First, there are *competitive sports* that pit two people against each other: tennis, handball, squash, and so on. Then there are *team sports* that can be adapted to more playful versions for two, such as football, volleyball, and basketball. And there are *solo sports* that you can do essentially side by side: swimming, surfing, water-skiing, running, cycling, and so on.

We've had fun with almost all of these sports, but when we started exercising together, we found that each kind of sport has its own advantages and disadvantages for two people who want to do it together. The competitive sports are great if you're both at about the same level of competence. But if you're not—as we weren't—it can be boring for one of you and frustrating for the other.

"Team" sports for two can be fun as long as you're just playing around. If you want to keep it up long enough for it to be beneficial, you'll probably need other people to form real teams to keep the contest even. Solo sports are great exercise, but you can't get really involved with the other person. You may be *with* the other person, running or swimming or cycling beside them, but you're not really interacting with them. Besides, if you go at it hard, one person may be left in the other's dust (or wake).

To solve these problems, to make aerobic sports easier and more enjoyable for *both* of us, we often try one or more of the following techniques.

Handicapping. When we play a sport together, whether it's tennis or beach volleyball, we use a system of handicapping, much like that used in golf, to give our competitiveness a real edge. For example, when we go to the pool, Jeff—who was a competition swimmer—swims two laps for every lap that Nancy does. Regardless of the sport, it doesn't take long for you to gauge your level of proficiency to your partner's so that both of you are encouraged to exert yourselves fully.

Intervals. Interval training can make your outdoor activity more beneficial to your heart and lungs. In interval training, you alternate periods of exercise and rest in a fixed ratio. For beginners, it should be one to one. For example, instead of jogging or swimming or cycling at the same speed for varying

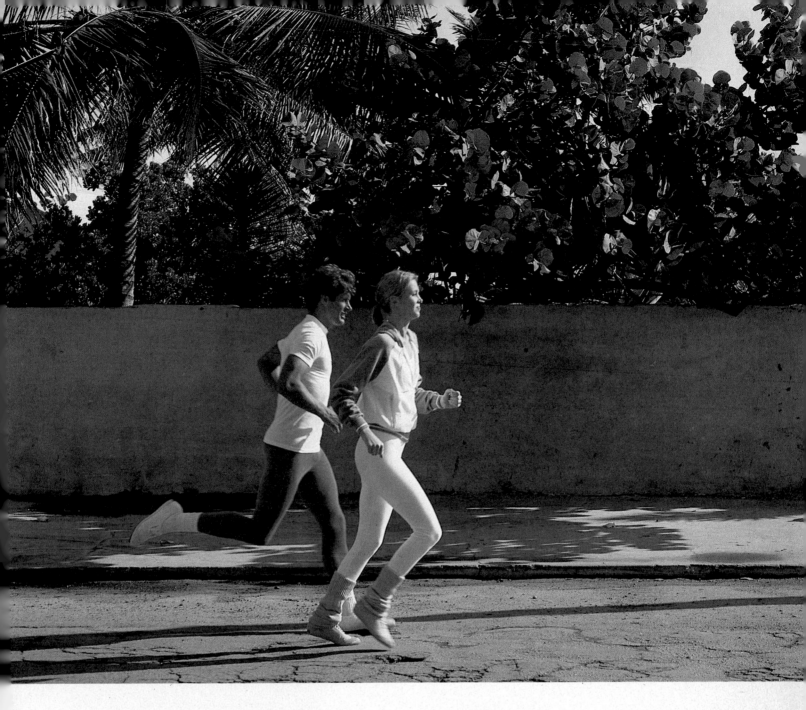

durations, you go at a greater intensity for a limited time, usually two to three minutes, then you slow down or even rest. Interval training is especially useful when two people are at different endurance levels—as we are—but want to work out together.

Timing. Another method we sometimes use to involve each other is to time each other. Keep track (even if only in your head) of your partner's best time and occasionally encourage him or her to beat it. That way, if you must compete, you're not competing with your partner but with yourself, with your own best time. Timing is especially appropriate if you're doing interval training. Sometimes, when we jog around a track or swim laps in a pool, one of us will jog or swim the lap while the other takes the time. Then we will switch places. (It's easy to compensate for greater strength or endurance by varying the number of laps.)

Contact. We don't mean "contact" as in "contact sports." We mean contact as in touching. A lot of sports aren't designed for touching, but, if you use your imagination, you can add that magic element. Whenever we get in the water together, whether it's a pool or an ocean, we end up very close: on a surfboard, a windsurfer, playing water polo, or just playing around. If you don't like touching someone else's sweaty body, you may not want to do much touching during strenuous exertion. Save it, as we often do, for the shower afterwards.

Motivation. The simple fact is that most people push themselves harder when someone is watching, encouraging them to do better. If you're a particularly competitive person and your partner isn't your competitive match, you can take turns sitting it out and providing vocal encouragement from the sidelines. Reaching your limit is easier when there's somebody else there pushing you toward it. But you should also consider the motivational power of *enjoyment*. Even if you are the competitive type, try to break the competitive habit by exercising for the fun of it occasionally. Not every activity has to be scored. Not every workout is a test. Instead of encouraging each other to do it faster, higher, longer, or better, try encouraging each other to enjoy it more.

AEROBIC DANCE

Aerobic dance is just one of the many forms of aerobic exercise. Like the others, its purpose is to develop your cardiovascular endurance by exercising your heart. The advantages of aerobic dance are familiar to most people in the Jane Fonda era. It improves your circulation, helps you breathe more easily, tones your muscles, improves your posture, reduces your appetite, and burns off calories (about three hundred per forty-five-minute session). Aerobic dancing can be done at home, it doesn't require a court or a track or special equipment, and almost anybody can do it.

Besides, when done to a heavy beat, it can be fun. Carol Hensel, an early advocate of aerobic dancing, says, "Many people view exercise only as a means to an end. They start a program for all the right reasons, then become bored with it and eventually drop out. Aerobic dancing is such a fun way to become fit that you can almost forget that you're

working out because at the same time you're enjoying yourself."

An aerobic "dance" is any combination of body movements that gets your heart rate up to the necessary level (sixty to eighty-five percent of your maximum) and keeps it there for the necessary

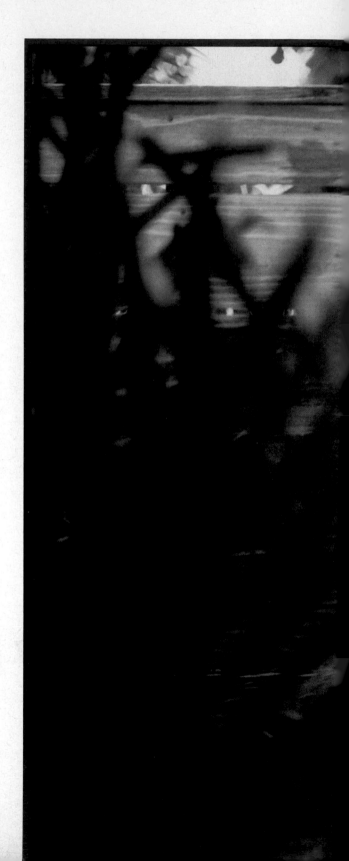

time (fifteen to thirty minutes). The same rule applies to aerobic dance as applies to any of the other aerobic activities we've already mentioned: It's more enjoyable and more effective if you do it together. You can bring to aerobic dance the same principles of cooperation, motivation, and physical contact.

If you already do aerobic dance, try the same thing we did: Take your favorite routine and figure out a way for two people to do it together. Invent a new routine that coordinates your movements. Here are a few simple ideas we use for turning common aerobic moves into dances for two.

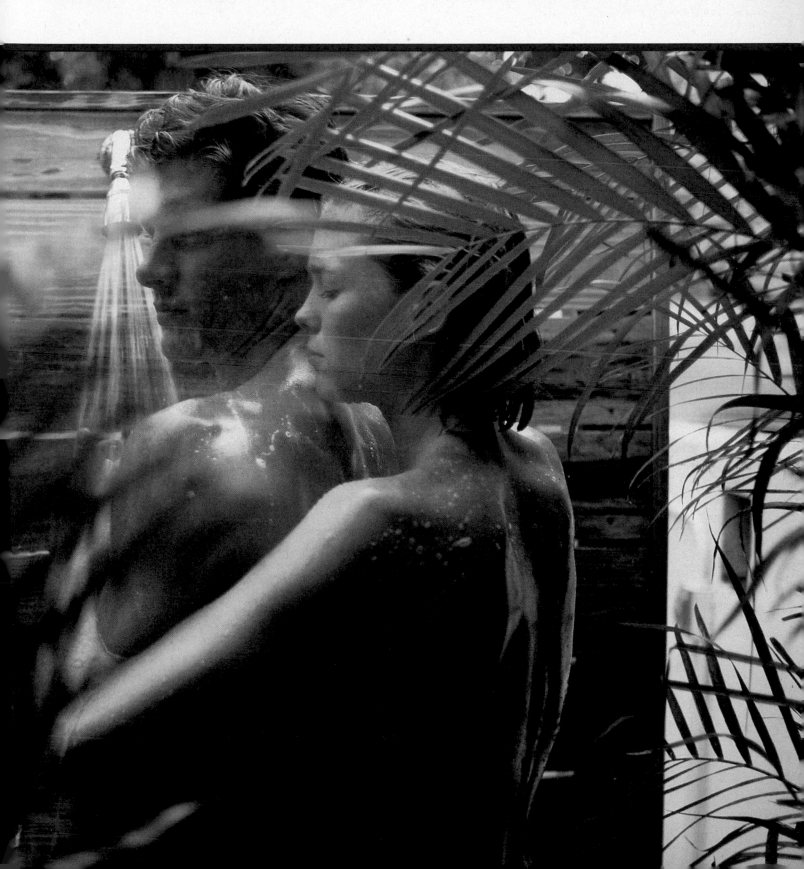

Chorus Line. Common aerobic kicks such as a can-can or a knee-up can be done side by side as in a chorus line. For seated exercises, where your legs are extended, cross your inside legs to form a W. Move from side to side in unison.

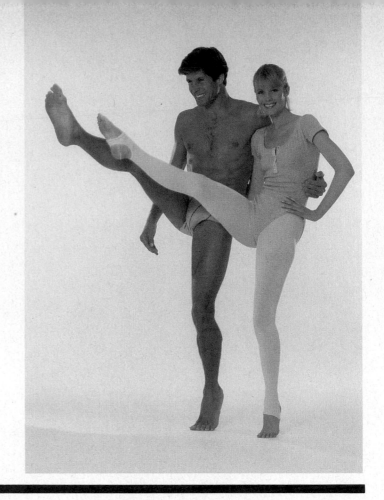

Single File. Line up behind your partner, both facing the same direction (pretend you're on stage and there's an audience out there). When you go one way, your partner goes the other. This is especially good for side reaches, side kicks, squatting side leg reaches, and so on.

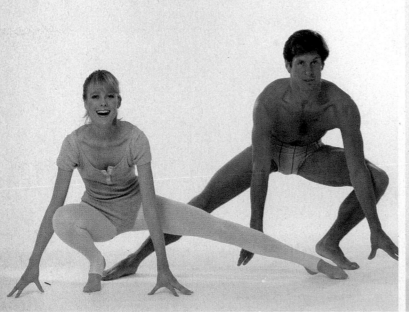

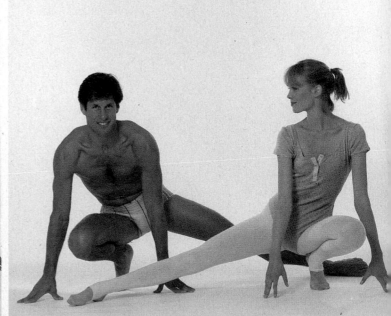

Face Off. When an aerobic step requires moving backward—push-ups, bridges, kick-backs, and so on—try facing each other. This position can also be used for sideways movements. Your motion can be together to the same side (as if in a mirror) or it can be a contrary motion (you go left when your partner goes right).

Rear-Ender. This is a good position for movements involving bending forward, bending down, or touching the floor. If you're standing and you bend down, make contact between your legs on each bend. If you're exercising while seated, sit shoulder to shoulder.

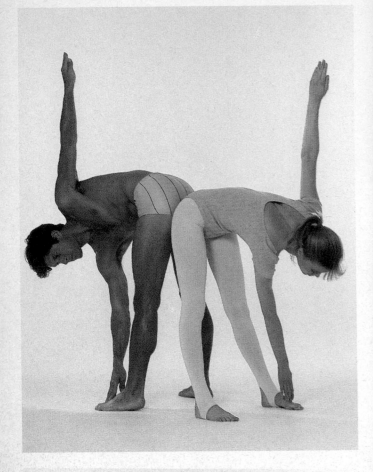

Arms-Length. For standing exercises, this position allows you to use your partner as a wall to lean on for treadmills and similar exercises. Keep your hands clasped and your arms straight, and come closer together into what we call a "tango hold," great for side reaches, hip isolations, and so on.

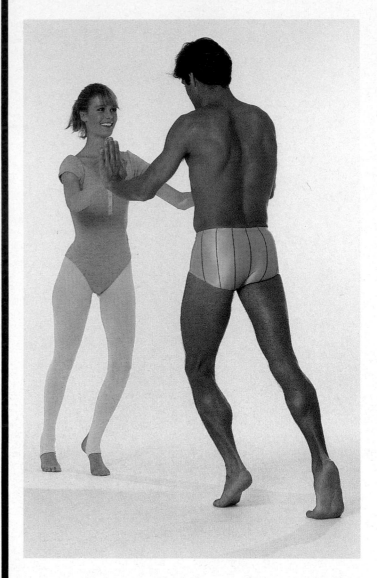

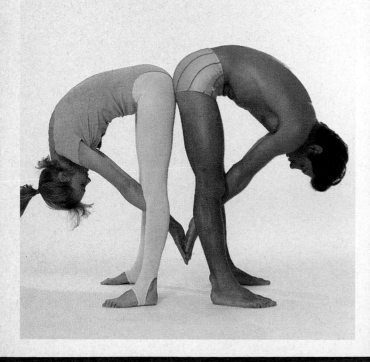

With a little thought and some improvisation, the advantages of doing it together—cooperation, contact, and motivation—can be brought to almost every kind of aerobic activity. Whether it's pacing each other on the track, alternating laps in the pool, or inventing a new aerobics routine, doing it together is more fun and better exercise. It's good for your body, and good for your relationship.

GENERAL ACTIVITY FOR A LIFETIME OF FITNESS

We believe that the best way to stay active is not to wait for specific opportunities, but to make your own opportunities, to incorporate aerobic activities into your everyday life. Both of us are amused to see the advertising executives we deal with running around the reservoir in Central Park. They huff and puff for a mile or two every day and seem miserable, but they wouldn't think of walking up stairs instead of taking the elevator, or of walking to that lunch date instead of taking a cab. If they weren't so lazy in their everyday lives, they wouldn't have to torture themselves around the reservoir every day.

A lot of people are in the same boat. They think that getting exercise is a separate part of their lives.

But in a truly active life, exercise is a part of living. It's riding a bike or walking to work if you can. It's forsaking the elevators, the escalators, the golf carts, the waiters, and the gofers, and using your legs. It's walking faster than you have to, carrying that bag rather than giving it to the porter at the airport or the bag boy at the supermarket. It's getting off the subway or bus one stop earlier or parking at the end of the parking lot instead of driving around endlessly trying to find the closest spot. The final piece in a complete exercise regimen is simply being active.

One of the great ironies of modern life is that we torment ourselves to make our lives so easy. Most of us expend too much mental energy trying to save ourselves a few steps. If only we could relax and walk the extra distance, we'd be much better off.

That's one reason why we live in a third-floor townhouse apartment in Manhattan—without an elevator. It's why we bicycle to studios and agencies around town when we could deduct the cab rides. It's why we go sailing rather than sunning at the beach. *Doing* things together—working, exercising, playing—is the best way to keep your body *and* your relationship fit.

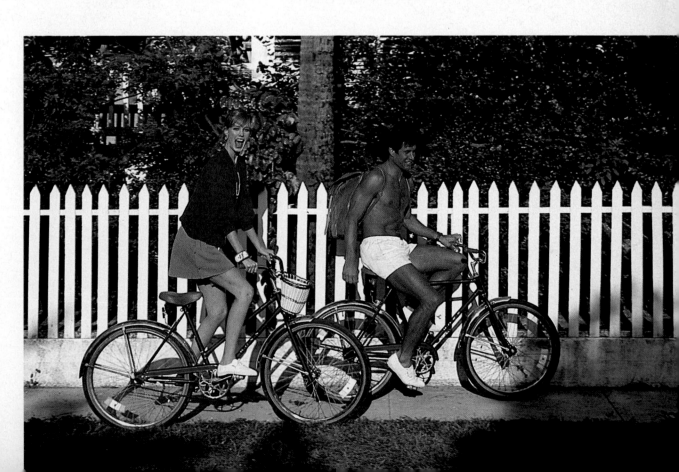

STEP FOUR/
Stress Control

COOL-DOWN AND MASSAGE

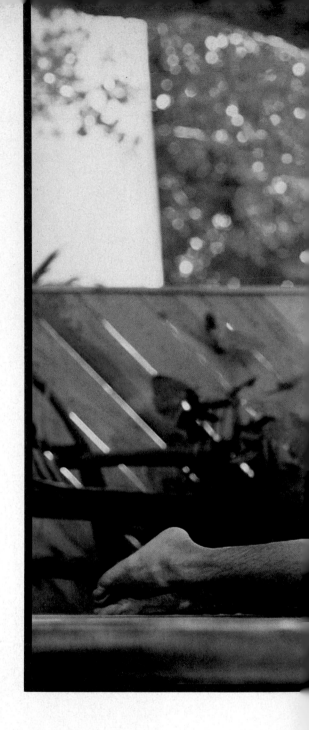

As models, stress is a part of our lives. The pressure and chaos of the "shoot" has sent many models into early retirement. But our lives are hardly unique. Stress is almost a universal phenomenon these days and most of us are ill-equipped to cope with it.

The failure to relieve stress can have serious effects, both short-term and long-term, on your body. Your heart, lungs, joints, and muscles are all adversely affected by residual tension in the body,

and the failure to work that tension out of your system can result in back pain, chronic headaches, arthritis, rheumatic pains, or high blood pressure.

Whether stress is the result of muscular exertion or office troubles, you should learn to control it through exercise. After a vigorous isokinetic or aerobic workout—or a hard day at work—it's essential to "cool down" with stretching exercises and massage. The goal is to relieve residual activity and tension in your muscles, to prevent pooling of

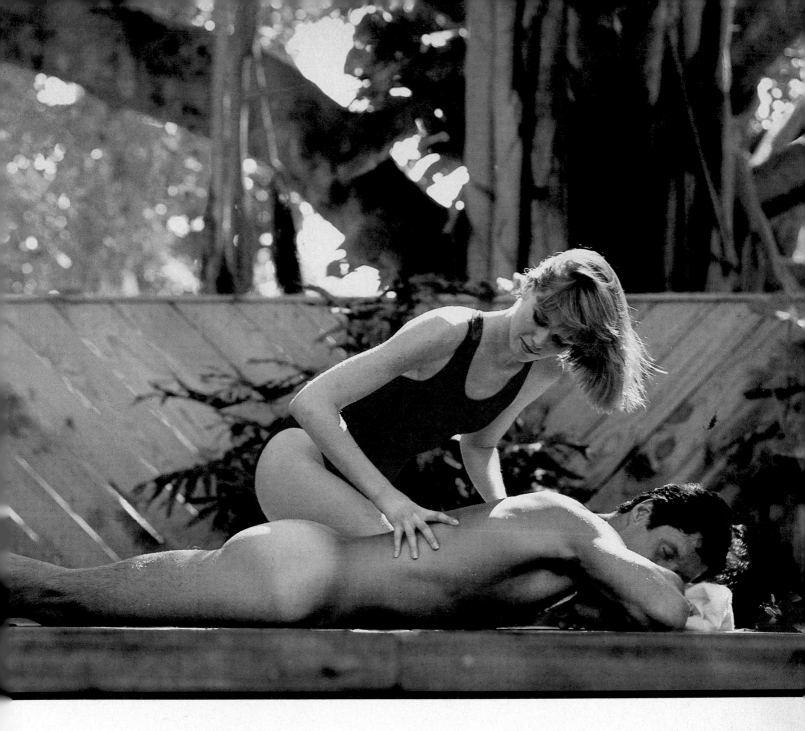

blood, especially in your arms and legs, and to promote general muscular relaxation.

The advantage of these cool-down exercises for two is that when you're the passive partner you don't have to work to stretch your own body. Most of the work is being done by the active partner. This allows you to relax more completely and to derive maximum benefit and enjoyment from the exercises. The advantages of doing it together in massage do not need elaboration.

COOL-DOWN EXERCISES

The cool-down routine should be done every time you work out, immediately after any isokinetic or aerobic exercise routine.

- Duration: Ten to fifteen minutes.
- Order: Sequences I and II, as shown.
- Repetitions: Two to three per exercise (each position, each partner) equals one set. Beginners and intermediates, do one set; advanced, two sets (four to six repetitions total).

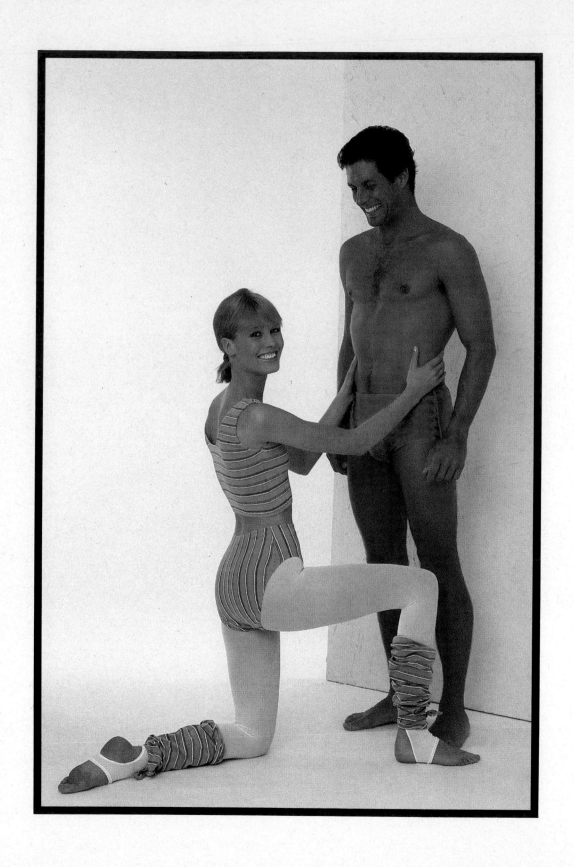

SEQUENCE I
#1 back, abdomen, hips

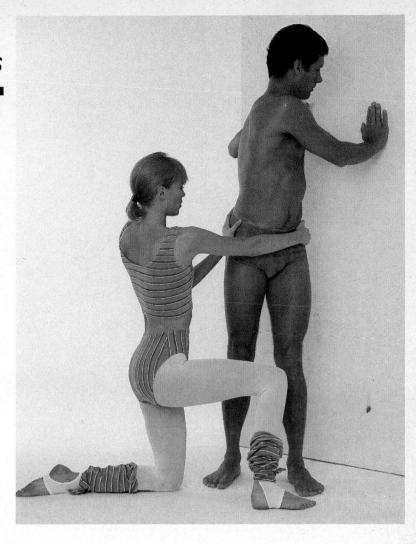

In these exercises, the passive partner is the one being stretched; the active partner is the one applying the pressure.

PASSIVE PARTNER:

Stand in front of a wall, facing forward, as shown. Without moving your feet, turn your upper body until you're facing the wall behind you. Put your palms against the wall at shoulder height and about shoulder width apart. Throughout the exercise, keep your feet and hands firmly planted and your face toward the wall. After one side is stretched, turn all the way around—feet still planted—and face the wall over your other shoulder and stretch that side.

ACTIVE PARTNER:

Turn your partner's midsection slowly toward the front by placing your hands on his hips and rotating the pelvis forward. Keep the pressure equal on both hips.

Passive partner, face the wall and sit on your feet.

SEQUENCE I   #2 *shoulders, arms*

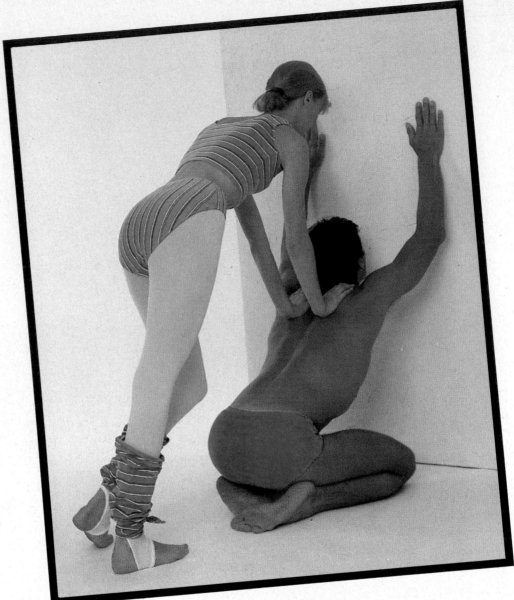

PASSIVE PARTNER:

Sit on your feet, facing the wall. Put your hands against the wall about shoulder width apart, as shown. Keep your elbows straight and your upper body relaxed (don't hunch your shoulders).

ACTIVE PARTNER:

Place your hands on your partner's upper back and gradually lean your weight downward. Make sure that the pressure is being applied through the heels of your hands, that the pressure is downward (not into the wall), and that your partner is not feeling any lower back discomfort (indicating that you're leaning too heavily).

Go back to the beginning of Sequence I and switch positions.

SEQUENCE II *#1 chest, shoulders*

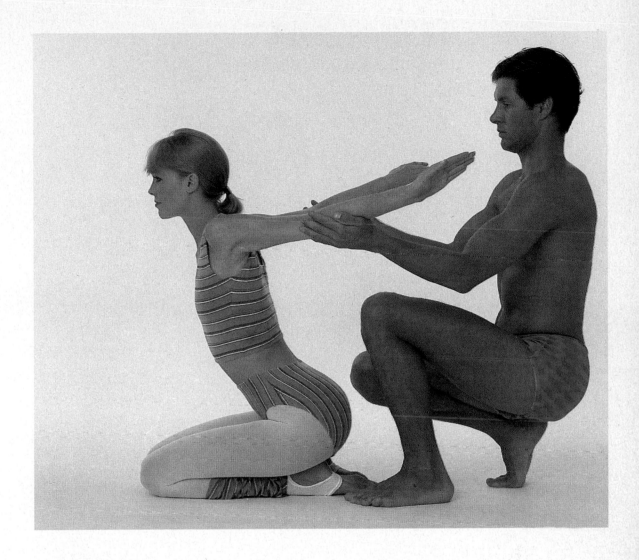

PASSIVE PARTNER:

Sitting with your feet tucked under you, as shown, stretch your arms out and back as far as you can. Keep your elbows straight and your shoulders relaxed. Your palms should be down or facing out. Spread your arms back to form a V no lower than shoulder high.

ACTIVE PARTNER:

Grip your partner's arms at the elbows and pull them slowly backward and upward. Proceed with care until your partner signals you to stop.

Passive partner, lie on your stomach.

SEQUENCE II *#2 thighs, hips*

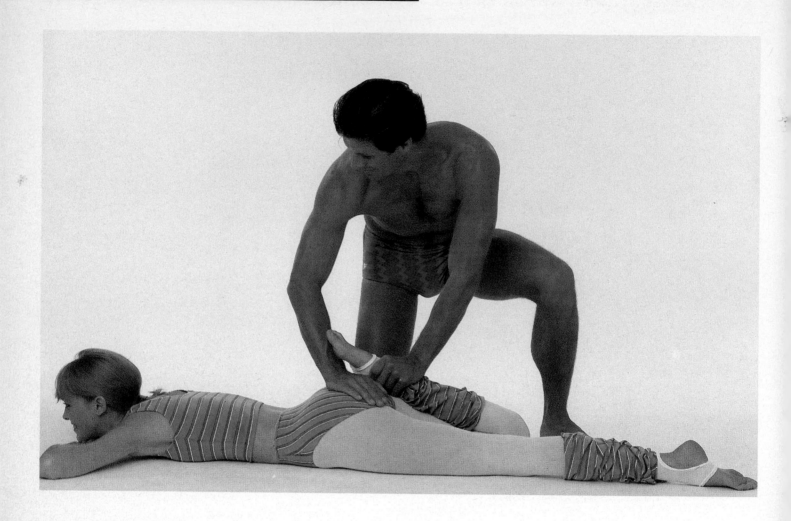

PASSIVE PARTNER:

You can lie with your hands at your side or under your chin. Assume whatever position is comfortable.

ACTIVE PARTNER:

To prevent your partner's hips from lifting off the floor and to maximize the stretch, hold the hips in place by pressing down gently but firmly on the upper part of the buttocks with the heel of your hand. With the other hand, lift your partner's leg, bent at the knee, and bring the heel of the foot as close to the buttocks as possible without pain. For some, this stretch will be effortless, for others it will take some practice before the heel can touch the buttocks comfortably. Repeat with the other leg.

Remain in the same positions.

SEQUENCE II #3 shoulders, chest

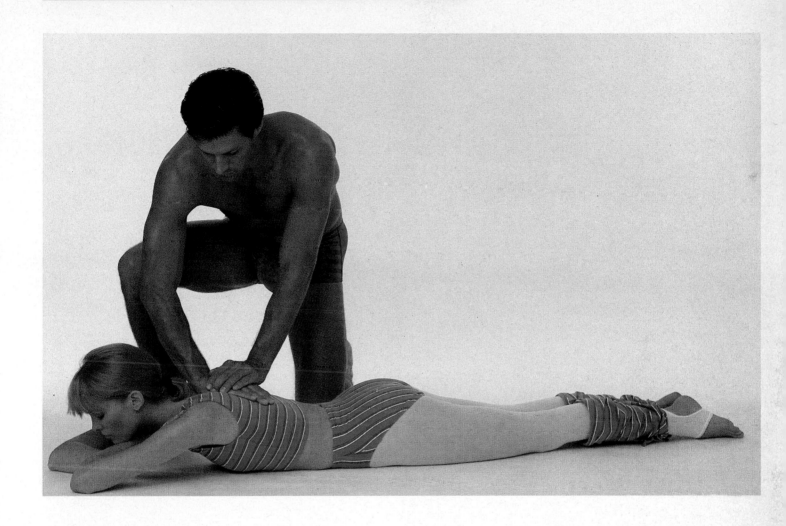

PASSIVE PARTNER:

Prop your head up by resting your chin in your hands as in the previous exercise. Remember not to hunch your shoulders.

ACTIVE PARTNER:

Put your hands on top of one another and press straight down on your partner's upper spine. Repeat several times at different spots if you like, coordinating your pressure with your partner's breathing. Watch for signs of discomfort.

Remain in the same positions.

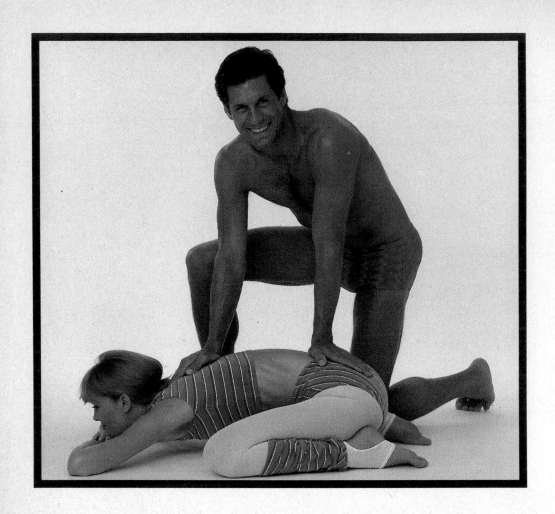

SEQUENCE II *#4 thighs, hips, buttocks*

PASSIVE PARTNER:

Cross your arms and rest your head on the back of your hand. Bring your knees up on both sides of your body until your heels touch your buttocks, as shown. It's all right if your lower body lifts off the floor as you bring your knees up. Keep your shoulders down and try to relax.

ACTIVE PARTNER:

Place one hand at the base of the spine (the sacroiliac) and the other at the highest point on the upper spine. Keeping your arms as straight as possible, gently but firmly lean your weight through your arms. The direction of your pressure should be down and backwards, toward your partner's feet. Apply more pressure to the hand nearest the feet. Increase the pressure only gradually. Let up a little when your partner inhales and increase the pressure when she exhales. The stretch in the thighs can be very acute.

Passive partner, roll over on your back.

SEQUENCE II *#5 hips, thighs, hamstrings*

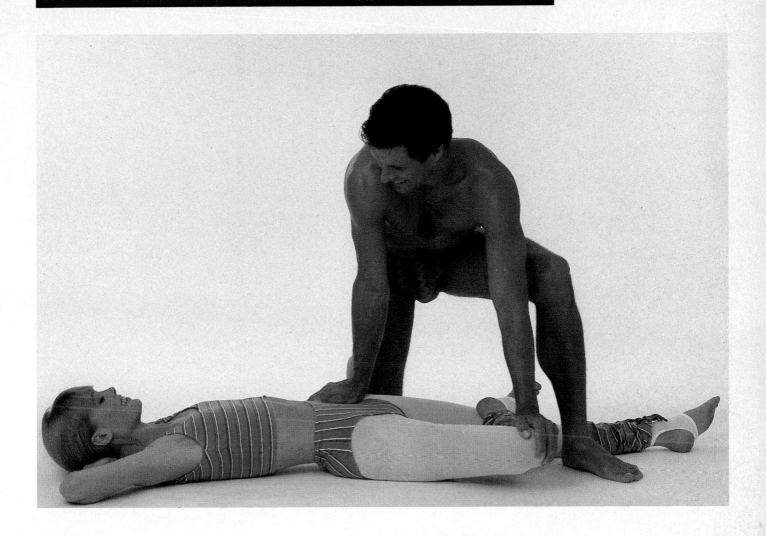

PASSIVE PARTNER:

Put your hands behind your head and get comfortable. Bring one leg up and cross it over the other leg so that the ankle of one leg rests just above the knee of the other, as shown.

ACTIVE PARTNER:

To prevent your partner's hip from rotating and to improve the stretch, place one hand on the hip above the straight leg and press down firmly. Place your other hand on the inside of the bent knee and gradually lean your weight onto it. Slowly press the knee toward the floor while maintaining an equal pressure on the hip. The stretching sensation can be acute, so be gentle. Repeat with the other leg.

Active partner, straddle your partner.

SEQUENCE II *#6 thighs, lower back*

PASSIVE PARTNER:

Put your arms down at your sides about shoulder width apart. Bend one knee and bring your foot up until the heel touches your buttocks, as shown. Keep the other leg straight. If you have trouble assuming the position, have your partner help you. Stretch each leg separately.

ACTIVE PARTNER:

Place your hands on your partner's hip bones and lean your weight gradually onto them. The most important thing is to distribute the pressure evenly on both hips. You can use your legs to keep your partner's legs close together. This stretch can produce some acute sensations, so go slowly.

Remain in the same positions.

SEQUENCE II *#7 hamstrings*

PASSIVE PARTNER:

Bring your feet up as close to your buttocks as possible. Now spread your knees apart and put the soles of your feet together. Let your knees drop as far as they will go without letting your feet slide away from your buttocks. In this exercise it's important to keep your lower back pressed against the floor. To do this, keep your buttocks slightly raised. You can prop them up by sliding your clenched fists underneath or, if necessary, by using a small cushion.

ACTIVE PARTNER:

Place your hands on the insides of your partner's knees and very slowly lean your weight down, pushing the knees toward the floor. Prevent the feet from sliding away from the buttocks by bracing them with your knees. Keep your arms straight and direct the pressure straight downward. Don't expect your partner's knees to touch the floor right away. For most people, it takes weeks or months to reach this position. Never go past the point of discomfort.

Remain in the same positions.

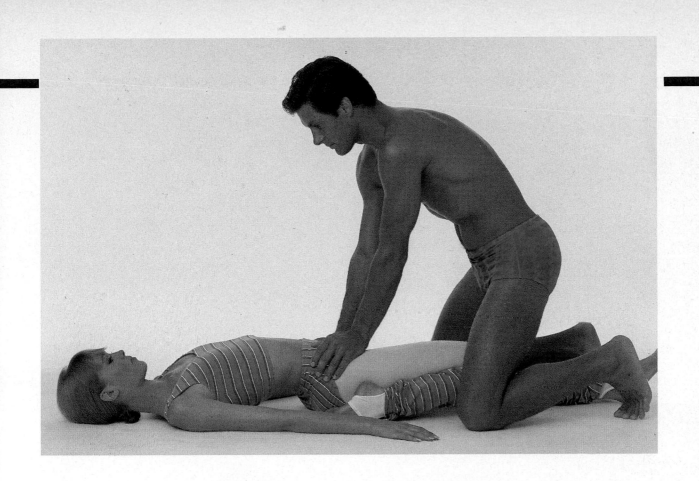

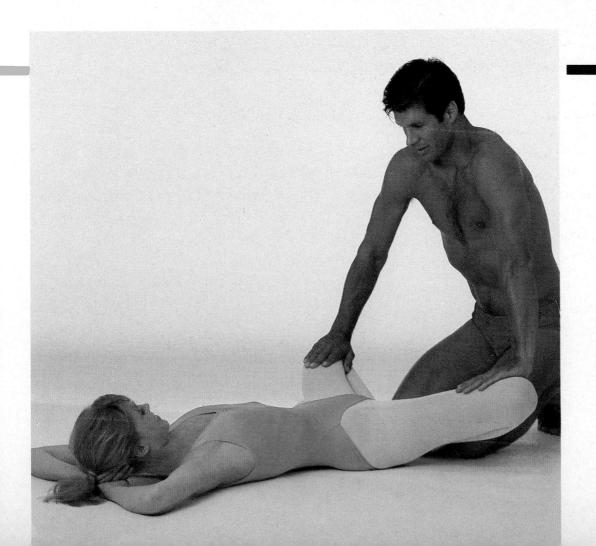

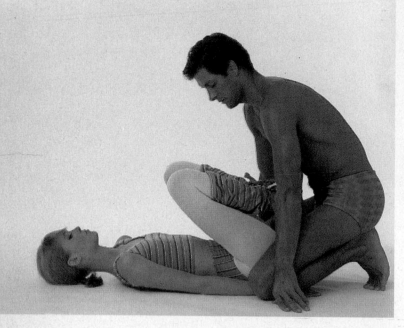

PASSIVE PARTNER:

Put your arms down at your sides and leave them there throughout the exercise. With your partner's help, roll your legs over your head until your feet touch the floor above your head.* Now lower your legs until your knees brush your ears and rest on the floor. If you can't bring your legs down this far, straighten them out so that only your toes touch the floor, as Jeff is doing on the opposite page. Hold this position for a few seconds. Eventually you will feel comfortable and will be able to hold the stretch longer.

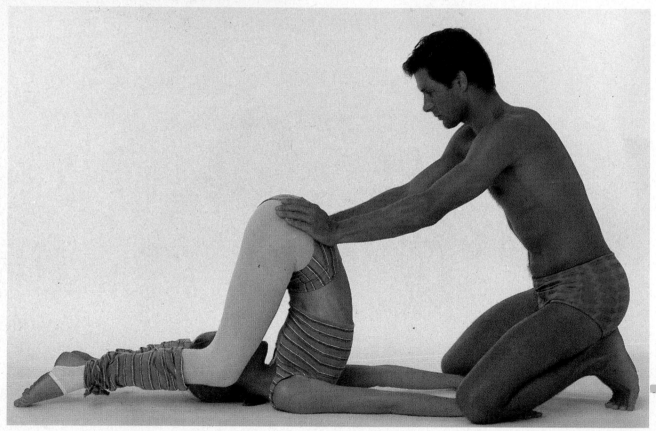

*If you're not able to assume either of the positions shown, begin the exercise with your head about three or four feet from a wall. When you roll over, plant your feet on the wall, legs together, and proceed with the exercise as described.

As you feel more comfortable in this position, begin the exercise progressively farther from the wall until it's no longer needed.

ACTIVE PARTNER:

Help your partner maintain her balance during the rollover. With your legs, anchor your partner's hands to the floor. With your hands, support your partner's lower back. Don't push much at all, unless your partner is very flexible. Many people who assume this position for the first time feel very insecure. The active partner's most important job is to provide the kind of physical and psychological support that will make this exercise a lot easier.

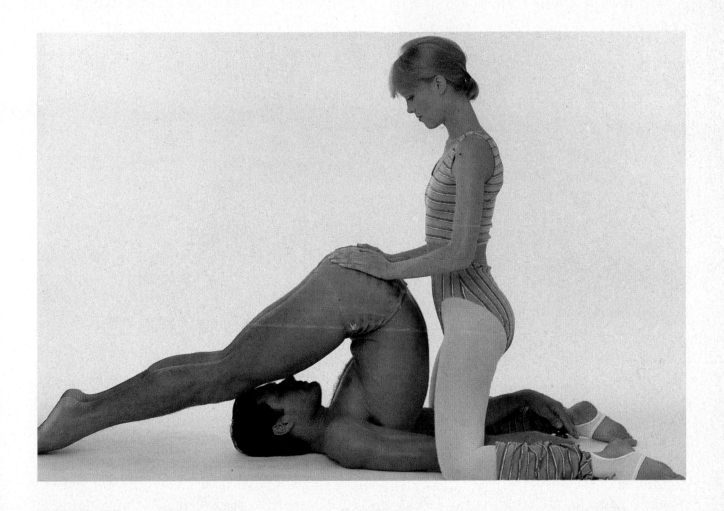

Go back to the beginning of Sequence II and switch positions.

MASSAGE

Another way that two people can control stress is by regular massage. Of all methods of stress control, massage is undoubtedly the most enjoyable. It's also great medicine for a relationship. We've found that working tensions and exercise soreness aren't the only things that melt away in the warmth of a good massage.

Different kinds of exercise require different massages. Swimming requires a relatively generalized massage because every muscle in the body is used. In some sports, however, one or more muscle groups are worked especially hard. For joggers, the most important muscles are the calf and thigh muscles. Tennis players will need more massaging in the shoulders and arms. Let common sense and sore muscles be your guide.

Of course, you don't have to restrict a massage to the sore areas. You can give sore areas extra attention as you massage the entire body. After all, the body is a unit that works together: If you release the stress and tension in one part of the body, but not the whole body, the other parts will remain tense and uncomfortable.

As enjoyable as it is, massage is much more than just a good feeling. Although it's certainly no substitute for exercise, it provides some of the same benefits, such as better muscle tone and improved circulation. It helps you "tune in" to your muscles. It makes you more aware of when you're becoming tense so you can control your tension more easily. It both reduces your *muscular* arousal level—so that you won't be as edgy, little things won't bother you as much—and, at the same time, increases your *sexual* arousal level.

In short, massage is good for your relationship as well as your body. After all, there's no better way for a couple to learn to give and receive pleasure. "You can't have an absent-minded, half-hearted massage," says Ouida West, a leading massage expert, "because your partner won't enjoy it." In massage, you both have to be able to give, and to let go and let the other person give to you. Massage is one part of fitness for which there is no solo version. It's either done together or not done at all.

To learn about massage, you should read *The Massage Book* by George Downing, *The New Massage* by Gordon Inkeles, *Loving Hands* by Frederick Leboyer, *Athletic Massage* by Rich Phaigh and Paul Perry, or *The Magic of Massage* by Ouida West, or ask the owner of your local health food store to recommend a legitimate professional masseur or masseuse.

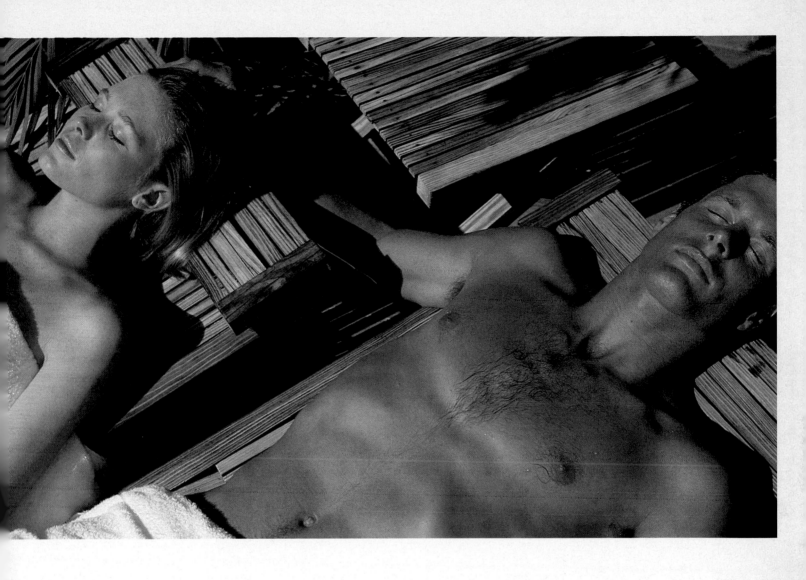

STEP FIVE/
Nutrition and Body Composition

THE "MODEL" DIET

Someone once said that a model who eats too much doesn't eat. That's undoubtedly true, but it's only part of the story. In fact, within the modeling community, certain models are notorious for their bad eating habits and indifference to nutrition. They eat erratically and irrationally: sneaking sweets, crash dieting, taking diuretics, and trying to compensate at the gym for the shabby way they treat themselves the rest of the time.

In other words, models are just like everybody else when it comes to diet and nutrition—maybe worse. They do manage to stay slim, for the most part, but they pay a high price to look so good. Because they can't binge-eat like normal people, they're even more prone to turn to alcohol or drugs if they're having emotional problems; and you don't need to be a doctor to know what effects addiction can have on even the most perfect body. We've seen many models who burned out after only a few years, largely because of the way they treated themselves. The "Model" Diet is no model diet.

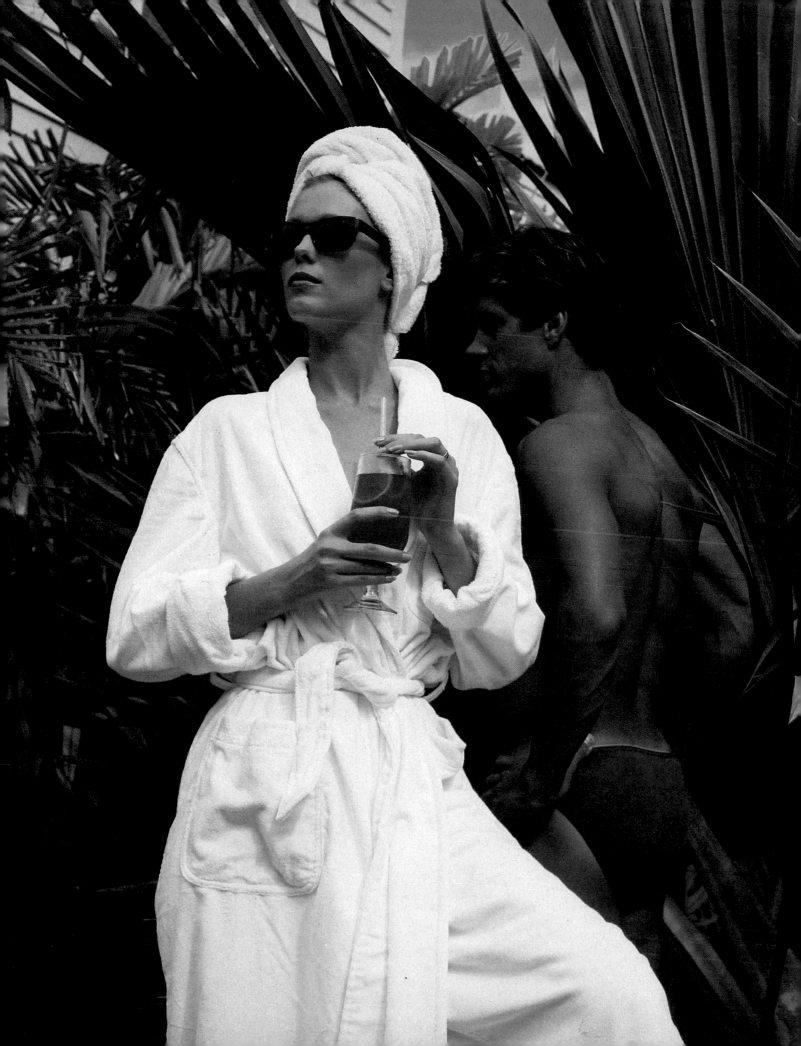

Jeff: Getting It Together. Of course, I suffered from the same pressures as any other model, and, for a while, I kept slim at my body's expense. The combination of a grinding schedule, irregular location shooting, and long periods away from home made a proper diet almost impossible. It also led to trouble when I was home because Nancy's schedule was not only overloaded like mine, it was also *different.*

Nancy still reminds me about the time I came home after a week-long shoot in Arizona with only one thing on my mind—a gallon of vanilla ice cream covered with fresh strawberries. I didn't have any jobs over the weekend, so I could afford to splurge. Nancy was scheduled to fly to Casa Marina in Key West the next day and shoot swimwear for Kamali. She'd been starving herself the whole week I was gone, but the first thing I did was go out and bring back ice cream and strawberries. She screamed in pain. I don't blame her; I would have been upset if she'd done that to me.

Nancy: Putting an End to Fads. Like most people— and almost all models—I have tried lots of diets. Especially among female models, there's always some fad in the business. At one time, for instance, there was a herbalist, a natural healer, many of us went to. He gave us thirty bottles of herbs and we'd carry them around with us all day. At appointed times we'd take ten drops of this and ten drops of that. After that, a vitamin fad took over and soon we were all taking the vitamins.

After suffering through a variety of these "snake-oil" diets, I decided to stop dieting and start thinking. I realized that if I ate right and exercised right, I could make dieting a thing of the past. Now the only time I consider dieting is in January and February. That's when the fashion industry photographs summer clothes and I have to look good in next season's swimsuits (see, in the next chapter, "Thirty Days into a Swimsuit").

We had different reasons, but we both finally came to the same conclusion: Eating right, like exercising right, is something that's a lot easier if you do it together.

What does it mean to "eat right"? First, it means recognizing your own weaknesses and not expecting the impossible. We haven't completely eliminated *any* food from our lives. We still eat pizza and ice cream and cheese cake and all the other fattening stuff, but we follow two rules: Never go on a binge alone and never go on two binges in the same week. We found that if you're dieting together and one person goes off without the other, all sorts of resentments and guilt feelings result. So when we want to go out and stuff ourselves with some forbidden food, we make a major event out of it. It becomes a pleasure we share, not one we hide from each other.

The rest of the time, we watch what we eat—*and* we watch what the other person eats. When we decided to develop a nutritional program for two, we both took the time to learn something about food. In the process, we discovered some interesting facts about nutrition that we didn't know:

- You should *not* cut fats completely out of your diet. If you're young, they promote body growth. For everybody, they contribute to healthy skin. Certain forms of fat are better than others, however, because they are more easily absorbed by the body. Olive oil and peanut oil (which is in peanut butter) are okay. Butter is taboo.
- You don't have to bar red meat entirely from your menu. An occasional steak or hamburger is pardonable. But because red meat is so high in taboo animal fats, it makes an appearance on our table about as often as red caviar. Another no-no is salt.
- Just as there are good and bad fats, there are good and bad carbohydrates. "Good" carbohydrates are found in vegetables, fruits, beans, and cereal grains. "Bad" carbohydrates are primarily the refined sugars found in candy and other sweetened products.
- Snack on protein. Proteins should account for at least twelve percent of your diet. Because the body doesn't retain protein as it does fat, you have to replenish your supply every day. For the same reason, protein makes an excellent snack as long as it's not a protein source that's high in fat, like meat.

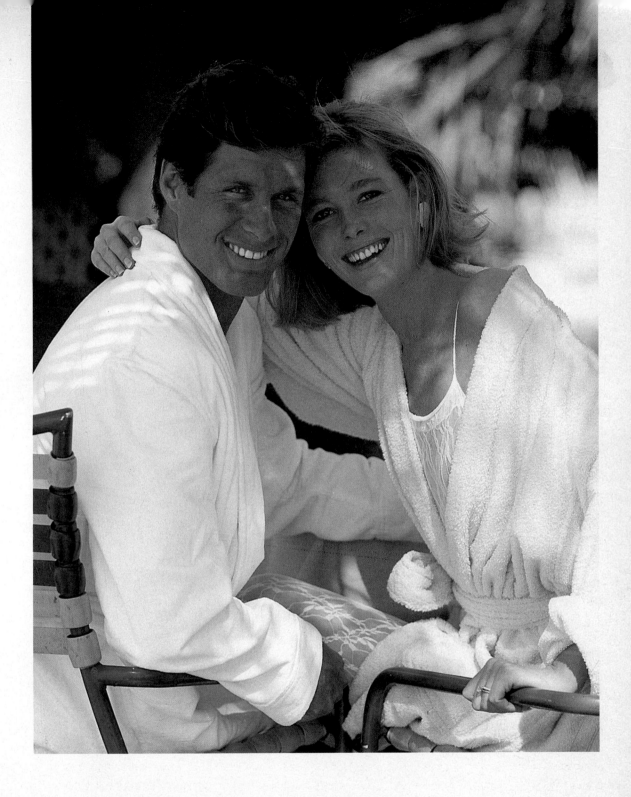

- Sugar is addictive. Surprise. We don't mean that it's easy to like. We mean that it is *literally* addictive, like nicotine or alcohol. Sugar gives you a temporary high followed by sluggishness and depression. We think of sugar like booze: It's a party food, great for special events with friends. But you don't drink champagne for breakfast.

- Never eat fats without eating carbohydrates at the same time. Carbohydrates make it easier to burn up fats. Don't eat fats just before or after exercising. Fats slow down digestion and the absorption of water. Also, get in the habit of drinking water before, during, and after exercise, especially in hot or humid weather.
- Avoid overprocessed foods. The further it is

from being plucked from a tree or pulled from the ground, the more it's been pummeled, processed, and wrapped by some giant food combine, the less of its nutritive value remains.

For us, eating right hasn't meant giving up our cravings for certain foods; it's meant training our bodies to have the *right* cravings. We used to get sugar cravings because we had altered our systems and become addicted to it. Once we had readjusted our bodies, they began sending out the right messages. Now, instead of telling us that we need an extra scoop of chocolate–chocolate chip ice cream, they tell us that we haven't had fresh fruit in twenty-four hours.

Your goal should be to internalize good eating habits, to get to the point where you don't need to sit down and make lists of your daily diet. After all, eating should be a pleasure. If you pay attention to what you eat long enough, your body will begin to tell you when you have strayed from good nutrition sense. The simpler you keep your diet the faster you'll be able to internalize it.

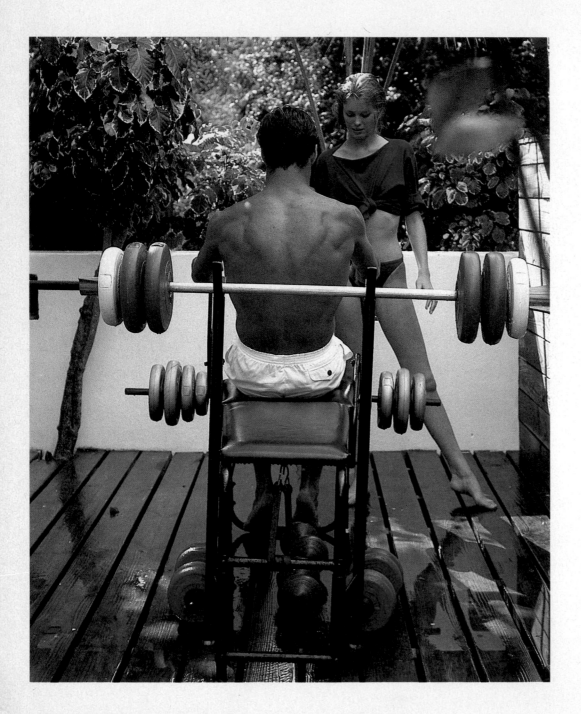

Diet, Exercise, and Body Composition. If you need to *lose* weight, eating right may not be enough. But dieting, by itself, is still not the answer. Most people think you should diet in order to reach a desired weight. In fact, there is fallacy behind "weight watching." You shouldn't be watching your weight, you should be watching your fat-to-muscle ratio.

Unfortunately, we all tend to watch the scale, because it's the only measuring device we have, even though what we really care about isn't our weight, but the amount of *space* we occupy. If you increase the amount of muscle in your body and decrease the amount of fat, you may weigh the same, or even more, but you'll occupy less space. You'll be able to fit into that swimsuit.

So keep your eye on the right goal—a better fat-to-muscle ratio. One of the ways you can do that is by getting rid of the bathroom scale. Instead of the scales, use "body calipers" as a way of measuring fat-to-muscle ratio. These are plastic devices shaped like small pincers that can be purchased (average price, ten dollars) from many exercise and health food shops. Directions accompanying the calipers will tell you where to take the measurements (usually shoulder, midriff, and thigh), and how your figures compare to "ideal" ratios for someone your age, height, and build.

The other rule for reshaping your body by improving your fat-to-muscle ratio is *Never diet without exercising at the same time.* That "doughnut" around the middle—the model's nightmare—is your body's reserve fuel, your own personal oil glut. To get rid of it, your body has to use it up. In weight loss, there's no such thing as spot removal. People who follow fad diets are fooling themselves. Even more important, they're *hurting* themselves. Of course, they aren't providing themselves with the nutrition they need. But they may even end up gaining weight instead of losing it.

All of us know the pattern: We go on a crash diet, starving ourselves for a week. We may lose a few pounds, but the minute we go back to eating regularly we gain it right back. Sometimes we even gain some more. After a week of self-inflicted torture, we end up looking worse than we did before we started.

To burn up that fat, you need to increase your body's metabolism. Someone with a fast metabolism can lose weight faster than someone with a slow metabolism and can eat more without gaining weight. The only way you can affect your metabolic rate is by changing your level of activity. Exercise tends to *increase* your metabolic rate; dieting tends to *decrease* it. That's why exercise is so important—more important than ever—when you go on a diet.

Here's how it works. When you just diet, you slow down your metabolism and your body tends to *conserve* energy, that is, fat. If you're not exercising, your body will lose weight it doesn't need: Some of the weight you end up losing is muscle, not fat. If you go off your diet, your slowed-down metabolism can't burn up the food, so you end up putting on fat. Unless you exercise, the net result of most diets is that you replace muscle weight with fat weight, your fat-to-muscle ratio goes to hell, you occupy more and more space. In short, you become another victim of middle-age spread.

A Pound a Week. To achieve the right muscle-to-fat ratio—and therefore the right weight—you need to attack the problem from both ends: Eat less and exercise more. By limiting the number of calories you take in and increasing the number of calories you burn up, you'll lose weight faster without having to starve and you'll be doing your body a favor. Also, exercise tends to suppress your appetite, which makes cutting calories even easier.

Here's a simple way to think of the relationship between exercise and diet, which we've worked out with the help of some experts. Every pound you want to lose represents about 3,500 calories. That means to lose one pound, you'll have to reduce your diet by that number of calories or you'll have to burn up that many additional calories. We suggest you go half and half. If you want to lose a pound in a week, that means 500 calories per day. Lose half of that, 250, by reducing your caloric intake and half by increasing the number of calories you burn up in exercising.

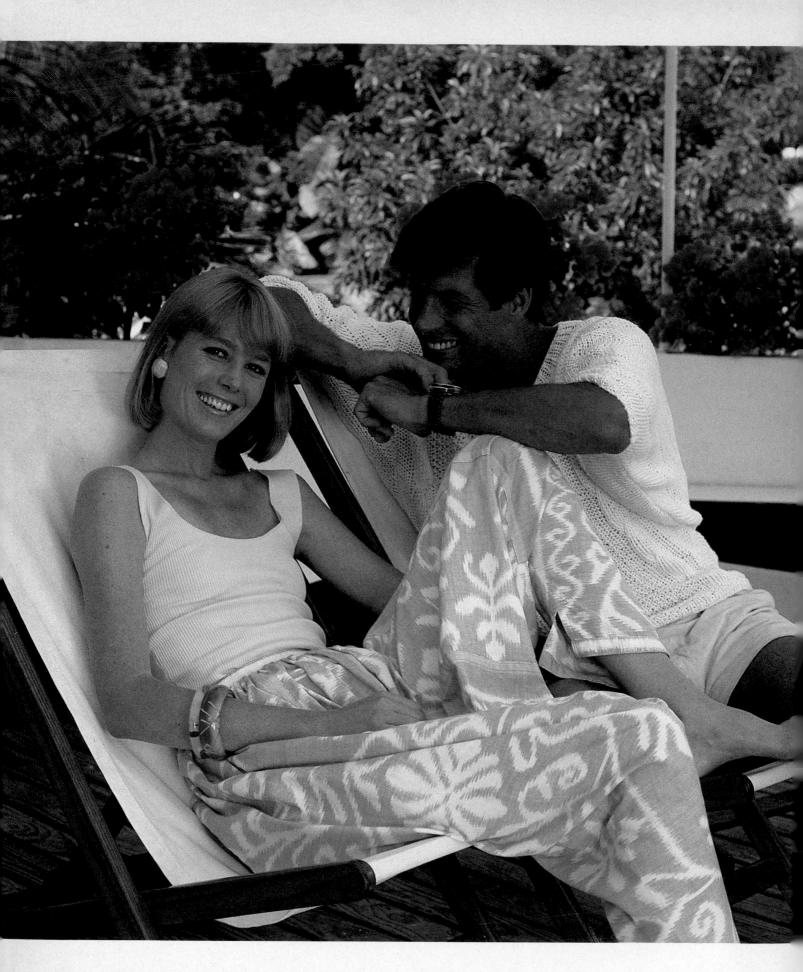

To help you know how many calories you're burning up when you exercise, here are some calorie values, according to body weight, for fifteen minutes of various kinds of exercises.*

BODY WEIGHT	110 pounds	150 pounds	190 pounds
Jogging (*slow*)	125	170	210
Jogging (*fast*)	200	265	330
Swimming (*breaststroke*)	120	165	210
Swimming (*crawl*)	95	130	165
Tennis	80	110	140
Aerobic dance (*slow*)	80	105	135
Aerobic dance (*fast*)	100	140	175
Isokinetic workout	140	190	240
Carpet sweeping	35	50	60

Motivation. By far the greatest advantage to eating and exercising together is the added motivation.

*These values are adapted from *The High Energy Factor*, by Bernard Gutin (New York: Random House, 1983). In the appendix to his book, Dr. Gutin, of Columbia University, has assembled "approximate energy expenditure" values for an extensive list of activities from sports to playing the piano to woodworking.

Eating right is partly a matter of the right foods in the right quantities with the right exercise, but it's also a matter of motivation. The hardest part of any regimen is sticking to it.

With the right motivation, almost any diet can be effective. Diet books can tell you what to eat and what not to eat, but they can't peer over your shoulder when you open the refrigerator. They can't follow you to the supermarket and hurry you past the doughnuts. They can't distract you with a joke in a moment of weakness. They can lead you to water, but they can't make you diet.

In our years of modeling, exercising, and dieting together, we've learned a lot about mutual support and setting examples. Whether we're cooking for one another, buying the groceries together, or eating out, we've developed a routine of reinforcement—a way to keep "diet motivation" alive with little comments like, "The good life's getting to you," or "You're a real New Yorker now."

Jeff will come to Nancy's rescue when she wants to stop off at a McDonald's.

Nancy will clear her throat when Jeff wants to indulge in a quart of Haagen-Dazs.

We've become each other's consciences, the little voice inside that says, "You know, you really shouldn't. You'll regret it later." It's much harder to ignore that voice when it's coming from someone sitting across from you, someone who cares about how you look and how you feel, someone you love. When it comes to dieting, two consciences are better than one.

THIRTY DAYS INTO A SWIMSUIT

Wearing swimsuits is part of what we do for a living. Because summer clothing is often photographed as early as January, we spend most of our winter months by the pool or at the beach in warmer climates. As comfortable as that schedule may sound, it doesn't save us from the usual trauma associated with walking around scantily clad in public. We just start worrying about it in the fall rather than in the spring. Of course, we try to swim all year round, but doing some laps in a health club is not the same as parading around in a crowded pool area.

For most people, the trauma starts in April or May, on the first warm day of the year. First you think how wonderful it is that winter's over and the good weather's back, then you get a sudden tightening in the stomach—the same stomach that's been slowly spreading since you put away your swimsuit last September. Summer is approaching again. And summer means vacations by the pool; it means weekend sun-bathing; it means bikinis and tan lines and lingering looks from behind sunglasses.

In short, it means getting out from under those

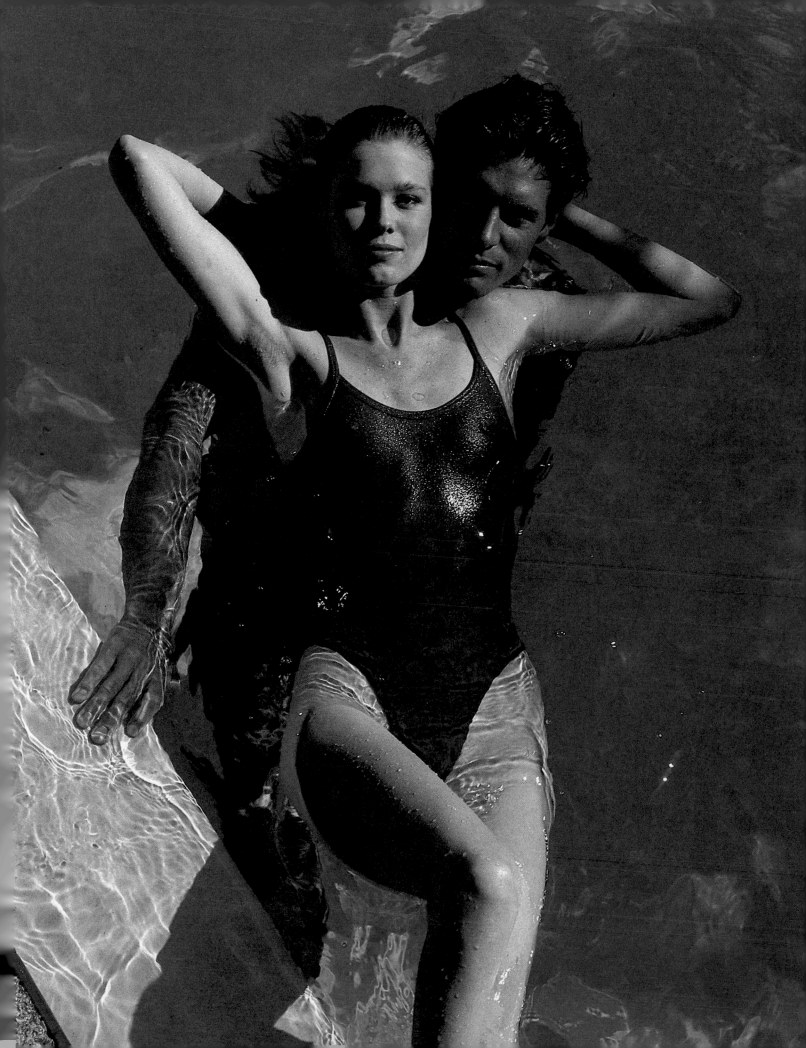

protective winter layers. The layered look has concealed and comforted you all winter long. When those layers finally come off, no wonder you feel naked and vulnerable. According to noted designer Norma Kamali, "Most women are afraid to stand nude in front of a mirror and try on a bathing suit because it forces them to see what they *really* look like."

There's no need to panic. Looking the way you want to look in a swimsuit doesn't take magic. Thirty days of exercising and eating right—and a better swimsuit—can transform that body you've been hiding into the body of your desire. To begin with, you probably don't need to lose more than about ten pounds. Typically, that's the difference between love handles and the body your partner would love to handle. And you have at least a month before your annual poolside debut.

Ten pounds in a month is, roughly, two and a half pounds a week. That won't require a starvation regimen; just more exercise and less food. If a pound of fat is 3,500 calories, that means you're aiming to rid yourself of 35,000 calories in about thirty days, or 1,200 calories per day.

All of that can't come out of your diet. Some people don't consume 1,200 calories in a day, and you have to eat *something*. That means that you're going to have to come up with a combination of reduced intake and increased output of calories that equals 1,200. The easiest thing to do is split the difference: Consume 600 fewer calories per day in your diet and burn off 600 more calories per day in your exercise.

First, you should calculate as exactly as possible how many calories you consume in an average day and how many you burn up. Figure that the average person sitting in front of the television or talking on the phone burns up approximately one calorie per hour for every two pounds of body weight. (When you're asleep, it's slightly less.) Therefore, a person who isn't active and who weighs 150 pounds consumes roughly 75 calories per hour or 1,800 calories per day.

Add to your "idling" figure the number of calories you burn off in your regular exercise routine. (Use the chart on p. 151.) If you do a half hour of jogging at a fair clip, add another 500 calories to the "burn-up" column. Most people burn up between 2,000 and 2,500 calories a day if they exercise a moderate amount, more if they're constantly on their feet or using their muscles a lot in their work.

In another column, add up the calories you consume in an average day. (Calorie counts for most foods can be figured from food packages and from cookbooks.) Typical daily consumption for someone not dieting is also between 2,000 and 2,500 calories.

To get into that bathing suit by June, you need to subtract 600 calories from the consumption column and add 600 to the burn-up column. What you do to reach this goal is your regimen for the next thirty days. You'll probably be surprised to find that it's not as demanding as the diets you've tried before. You should be able to consume over 1,000 calories a day, but you will have to dedicate at least another half hour daily to your exercise program.

Of course, if you need to lose ten pounds, chances are good that you haven't kept in shape and you're not doing as much exercising as you should. In that case, burning another 600 or more calories a day might mean stepping up—or even starting—your exercise program at too high a level. Running five miles, for example, would put too much load on your leg muscles. It would probably be better for you to distribute the additional exercise among several different activities.

Break up the additional 600 calories of activity into different muscle groups: Jog, swim, play a game of tennis, and do several sets of the isokinetic workout. Park your car a mile from work and walk the rest of the way or take a brisk walk at lunch. If all these activities aren't available to you—either because of the time or because of location—you may be forced to reduce your consumption of calories even further to make up for the exercise you're missing. Be flexible, but don't rob your muscles to pay your stomach.

The best thing about dieting this way is that it's relatively easy, and therefore you can stick with it. You don't have to do the impossible. Also, unlike most diets, it's adjustable. If you go off one day, you can make up for it the next. If you go out on a business lunch and eat too much, you know you have to exercise that much more that evening. If you have to stop exercising fifteen minutes too early one night, you know you have to cut your food intake the next day and you know how much you have to cut it by.

If you eat the right foods, you'll not only lose ten pounds, almost all of those ten pounds will be fat. Your contours will tighten, your muscles will firm up, and your fat-to-muscle ratio will improve. Unlike some diets that leave you feeling like you just weathered an illness, this thirty-day swimsuit shape-up will leave you in better health than when you started, and that perfect swimsuit will fit you perfectly.

THE PERFECT SWIMSUIT

After thirty days of eating right and exercising right, your body deserves a swimsuit that flatters it. Here are some guidelines, for both men and women, to help you find that "perfect" suit.

- Wait until you have finished your exercise/diet program and have achieved the *shape* you want (forget what the scale says).
- Choose the right fabric. If you plan to do more sunning than swimming, choose a cotton-Lycra blend. If you plan to spend hours in chlorinated water swimming laps, go for a nylon-Lycra blend instead. It won't pull out of shape.
- For comfort and resiliency, the suit should be tricot construction. You can tell a nylon suit is of tricot construction if it has good two-way stretch.
- A good swimsuit uses flatlock stitching: The

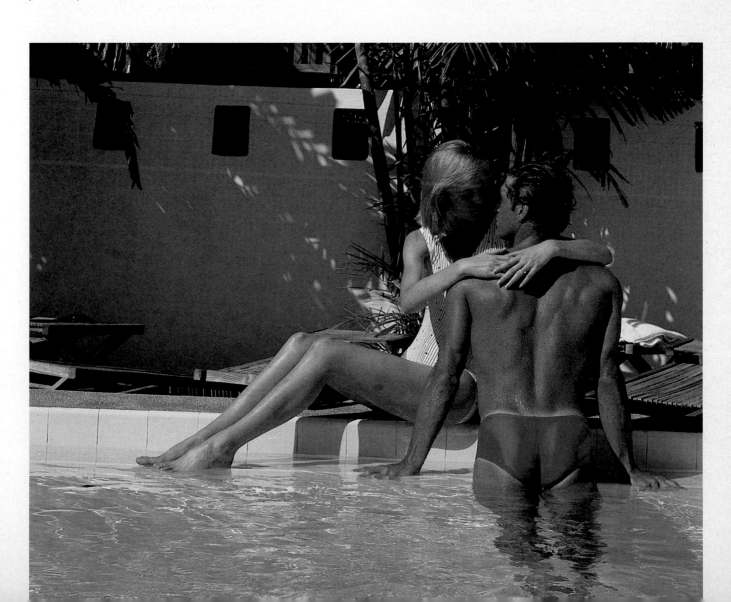

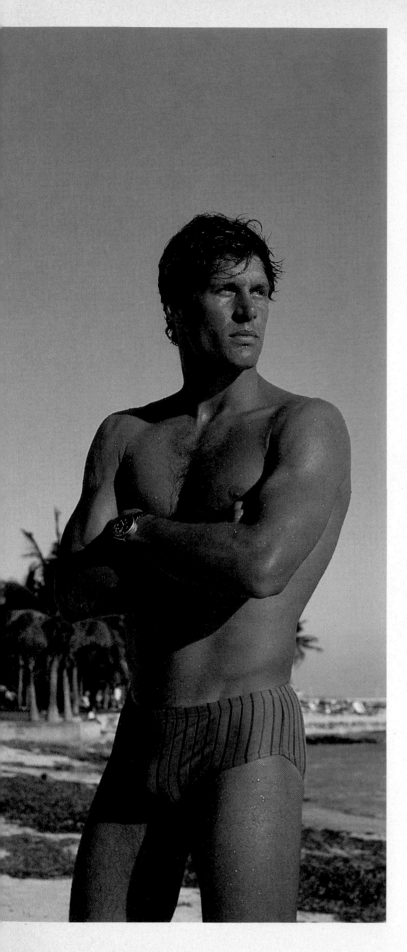

fabric is overlapped and the stitching shows on the outside so that it will lie flat against the body. Multiple stitching gives the suit needed stretch—also, if one thread breaks, the suit won't fall apart.

- The best leg hems are made of rubber, not elastic. The stitching on the inside of the hem should cover the rubber entirely so that the rubber won't chafe your skin.
- There should be a bar tack at every stress point (for example, where the strap on a woman's suit comes into the body of the suit).

Nancy: Hints About Swimsuits for Women. I should know something about swimsuits, I've worn at least a thousand of them since I began modeling. One-piece or two-piece; revealing or cover-up; rainbow-colored or basic black; I've worn them all.

But I haven't looked good in all of them. Even the best photographer can't change the facts of nature. Certain styles, cuts, and colors look better on some people than on others. For example, I look terrible in a "full-figured" swim suit. Bikinis may flatter a full bosom, but they also betray a small one. That's why I always wear a one-piece that's cut high on the leg, low in the front, and low in the back.

A new style of swimsuit that has recently become very popular, especially for sunning, is the kind with a thong bottom that can be worn without a top. "The smaller the suit," says Kamali, "the more popular it is. I think it has to do with how fit women are and the condition their bodies are in. Women of all ages are taking care of their bodies and looking terrific."

Other hints for helping you select the swimsuit that flatters your body best:

- On one-piece suits, a V neck makes your bust look fuller than a rounded neck. High-cut V legs make the hips look slimmer and the legs look longer and more shapely.
- Choose the best back for you by trying on several styles. Be sure the straps are comfortable when you raise and lower your

shoulders. If you move your shoulder blades and the straps don't shift, then you know you have a suit that's right for you.

- If a suit fits properly, there will be no rippling across a surface or gapping at the neck or back openings.
- Modesty or full breasts may argue for a constructed bra; this is basically a matter of personal preference.
- If you want to look slimmer, choose dark colors over light ones, and diagonal stripes over horizontal ones. Sheryl Page of Speedo also recommends "mitered stripes—stripes that miter into a seam down the center."
- If you're especially concerned about your thighs, consider suits with lighter colors at the top and dark colors at the bottom, or stripes that are narrow at the bottom and wider at the top (called the "sunburst" look).
- Vertical stripes can make you look thinner at the waist but they are not flattering on the hips. Horizontal stripes are great for the chest area but will add unwanted pounds to your hips.

Once you have found a suit that looks good on you, stick with it. Ignore annual changes in the fashion industry. "Maillots may have been very big last year," Kamali says, "and now everyone is going to want to be looking at bikinis, or vice versa. That doesn't mean you should too. A swimsuit is still a very personal purchase. Swimsuits don't go out of style, they really go on forever. Find a suit that's great for you, get it in a couple of colors, and let that be your summer signature."

Jeff: A Suit Is Not Just a Suit. It used to be that men's swimsuits came in one shape—full-cut boxer—and one size—too big. In those days, men didn't face the same perplexing array they face today, everything from the traditional baggy boxer to loincloths so skimpy they look more like G-strings.

When I swim, I always wear a tank suit (the kind you see on Olympic swimmers). When I went surfing as a kid, I always wore boxers. It wasn't until the tenth grade that I put on my first tank suit. I was horrified. To my untrained eye, it looked like underwear. Now I wouldn't wear anything else. Tank suits still seem strange to most Americans. They're still vaguely European. But there's no getting around the fact that they're infinitely better for swimming.

Although men don't have the range of choices women do in buying a swimsuit, there are some things to remember when you're looking:

- This may be a matter of personal preference, but I advise against bikini-cut swimsuits. Not only do they look silly and exhibitionistic, you can't swim in them.
- Tank suits are for men who have relatively taut stomach muscles and firm buttocks. Avoid them if you don't.
- If you're a little flabby around the middle, tight elastic at the waist of a suit will accentuate the problem.
- If your problem is "love handles," a boxer suit may accentuate them. Try a tank suit that is cut lower on your waist.
- If you have thin legs, a boxer-type swimsuit will only accentuate the problem. "More and more men," says Sheryl Page, "are becoming aware of what a tank suit will do for them."
- If you want to try a tank suit for the first time, go for a fuller six- or seven-inch cut rather than the skimpier three-inch cuts.
- Diagonal stripes look good on any man, just as they do on any woman. But vertical stripes work much *better* on men than they do on women.

The final test of the right swimsuit is simply what it looks like. When you set out to buy a new suit, take the opportunity to look at a wide range of styles and cuts to see which one looks best on you.

FEELING GOOD

Why do we care so much about exercise and nutrition? This may sound strange coming from two people who make their living on their looks, but looks is not the reason. Looks are important, of course, no matter what you do for a living. But looking better is not the best reason to eat right and exercise right.

When we meet people who aren't involved in the fashion world, they often think that a model's life takes place entirely on the pages of magazines, newspapers, and catalogs. They think we *always* look that way, that we're *always* in front of a camera. It's as if we live from shoot to shoot with no time in between for more mundane things like groceries, dishes, paying the bills, or feeding the dog.

In the pictures, we convey the impression that the most important thing in our lives is how we look. But that's not the case at all. Even though our careers *depend* on the way we look, we rarely *think* in terms of appearance. Sure, we worry about pimples or extra pounds, or cuts and bruises, but doesn't everyone?

What we do think about is being healthy and feeling good. We want to have a grip on our bodies. Instead of letting our bodies control us, we try to control our bodies so we can do the things we want and enjoy them. We don't exercise and watch our nutrition because our jobs require it. We do it because we care about how we feel. We know that if we aim toward health we'll end up looking better too.

Our experience in modeling has taught us that you *do* look better if you're healthy and fit. It's illusive to try to look good. You can never be sure when you've succeeded; it's hard to *know* when you look good. But it's easy to know when you feel good. So we try to keep fit because it makes us feel better. But there are other benefits too. One of them is that keeping fit helps us cope with the

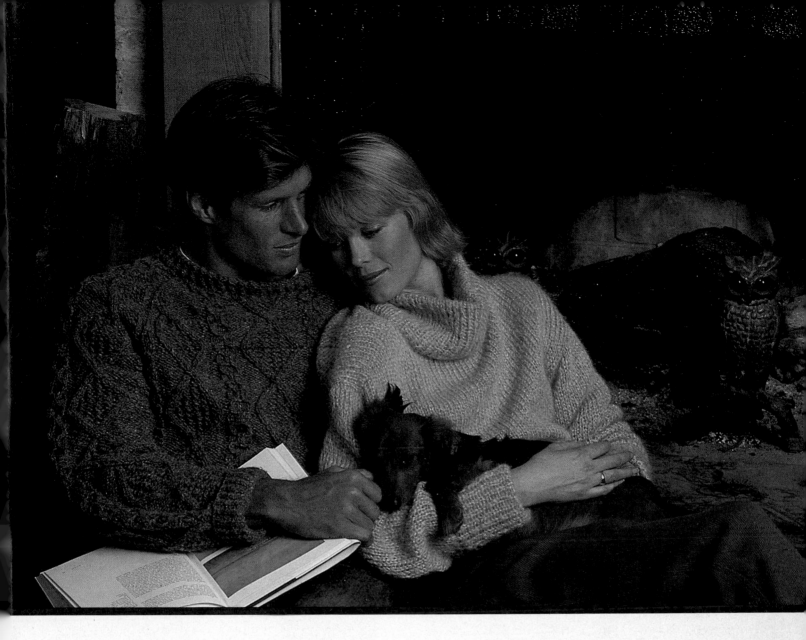

stress of daily life. Like many modern professions, modeling is hard work. There are many advantages to the career we've chosen. We've seen more of the world than we had ever thought possible. We've made many friends. And we've seen a fascinating industry from the inside.

But we've also spent long hours working with people who may or may not be congenial. We've eaten countless meals in third-rate restaurants, lost sleep on long plane flights, braved bitter cold in swimsuits, bundled up in furs in the summer heat, and put our heads down at night in strange hotels in places we can hardly remember.

Not surprisingly, it's become something of a private joke between us. Around Wednesday of every week, Jeff will say: "If I can just get through to the weekend..." But of course next week is usually just as hectic. At times like that, *looking* good doesn't help, but feeling good does. Whether it's the demands of a busy schedule or the ups and downs of a loving relationship, feeling good will make the lows more endurable and the highs more enjoyable.

That's the real payoff when you stay fit together. Feeling good about yourself makes it easier to feel good about each other. It enriches your relationship and rejuvenates your sense of romance. And, of course, once you feel good about each other, it's easy to feel good about everything else.

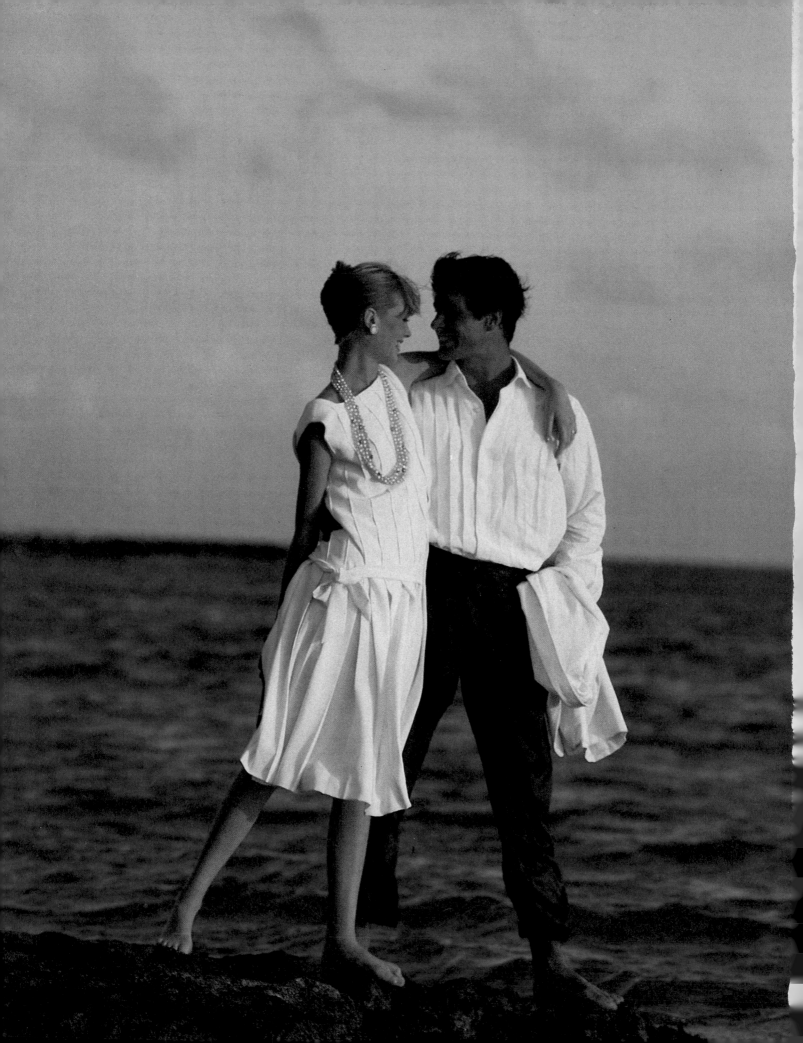